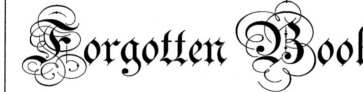

ISBN 978-1-330-35659-3
PIBN 10039125

1 MONTH OF FREE READING

at

www.ForgottenBooks.com

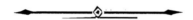

By purchasing this book you are eligible for one month membership to ForgottenBooks.com, giving you unlimited access to our entire collection of over 1,000,000 titles via our web site and mobile apps.

To claim your free month visit:

www.forgottenbooks.com/free39125

English
Français
Deutsche
Italiano
Español
Português

www.forgottenbooks.com

Mythology Photography **Fiction**
Fishing Christianity **Art** Cooking
Essays Buddhism Freemasonry
Medicine **Biology** Music **Ancient
Egypt** Evolution Carpentry Physics
Dance Geology **Mathematics** Fitness
Shakespeare **Folklore** Yoga Marketing
Confidence Immortality Biographies
Poetry **Psychology** Witchcraft
Electronics Chemistry History **Law**
Accounting **Philosophy** Anthropology
Alchemy Drama Quantum Mechanics
Atheism Sexual Health **Ancient History**
Entrepreneurship Languages Sport
Paleontology Needlework Islam
Metaphysics Investment Archaeology
Parenting Statistics Criminology
Motivational

THE NEWER KNOWLEDGE

OF NUTRITION

THE USE OF FOOD FOR THE PRESERVATION OF VITALITY AND HEALTH

BY

E. V. McCOLLUM

SCHOOL OF HYGIENE AND PUBLIC HEALTH, THE
JOHNS HOPKINS UNIVERSITY

ILLUSTRATED

New York

THE MACMILLAN COMPANY

1918

PREFACE

The need for knowledge of nutrition was never greater than at the present time when so large a part of the energies of the people of Europe and America are absorbed in the activities of war. The demoralization of agriculture over wide areas, together with the shortage of tonnage for the transportation of food, have reduced the food supply of a number of nations to the danger point, and have cut off in great measure the opportunity for securing the variety which exists in normal times.

The investigations of the last few years have, fortunately, led to great advancement in our knowledge of what constitutes an adequate diet. Such knowledge can, if rightly applied, greatly assist in enabling us to make use of our food supply in a manner which will avoid mistakes sufficiently serious to become reflected in a lowering of our standard of public health. It seems certain that pellagra is the sequel to the adherence to a faulty diet for such a period as to materially reduce the powers of resistance of the body to infection, and reasons are presented in support of the view that there is a much closer relationship between the character of the diet and the incidence of tuberculosis than has hitherto been believed. This view is offered in the present discussion as an invitation to criticism, in the hope that new data either in support or refutation of its validity will be presented. If it shall be definitely proven that faulty diet is the chief factor in the etiology of this disease, and that pellagra, is, as the Thompson-McFadden Commission, Jobling and Peterson and others believe, caused by infection, it will establish that, as the author suggests, large groups of people are at the present time making serious errors in the selection of foods. Regardless of the outcome of future studies relating to the importance of diet to the etiology of these diseases, a non-technical presentation of the kinds of combinations of our natural foods which induce good or faulty nutrition in animals, should be of service in showing the inadequacy of the practice, which is still in vogue, of regarding calories as the factor of prime importance in the planning of the diet.

From the data discussed in the following pages it will be evident that the idea that freedom of choice, and variety of food sources for the diet will prevent any faults in the diet from becoming serious, is no longer tenable, especially if one is willing to admit

the existence of many degrees of gradation of malnutrition, not recognizable except in their effects on
the individual óver a long period of time. The
author recently enjoyed with a friend, a dinner
which consisted of steak, bread made without milk,
butter, potatoes, peas, gravy, a flavored gelatin
dessert and coffee. The meal was appetizing and
satisfying, but such a diet of seeds, tubers and meat
would not promote health in an experimental animal
over a very long period.

The literature which has a bearing on the application of modern research to the practical problems
of human nutrition has become somewhat extensive
and is scattered in technical journals, and is not
readily accessible, or easy to read in proper sequence.
During the present year the author had the pleasure
of presenting an interpretation of this literature in
the Thomas Clarence Cutter Lectures at the Harvàrd
Medical School. Believing that the publication of
these lectures would serve to answer many of the
questions which have been asked in numerous letters
from the public, they have been edited and presented
in their present form.

It is a pleasure to acknowledge the author's in-
debtedness to those who have assisted in carrying
out the experimental work which made possible the

discussion of nutrition offered in this book. Nearly three thousand feeding experiments varying in length from six weeks to four years have been observed. Special appreciation should be accorded to Miss Marguerite Davis who assisted with the early work, in the first two years of which no interpretation of the cause of success or failure of our experimental animals was possible, and to Miss Nina Simmonds and Miss Helen T. Parsons for their keen interest and never-failing loyalty to the work.

E. V. McCollum.

The Johns Hopkins University
  School of Hygiene and Public Health,
    Baltimore, Md.

CONTENTS

CHAPTER   PAGE

I. THE BIOLOGICAL METHOD FOR THE ANALYSIS OF A FOOD-STUFF.................................. 1

II. EXPERIMENTAL SCURVY AND THE DIETARY PROPERTIES OF VEGETABLES................................. 34

III. THE VEGETARIAN DIET.......................... 53

IV. THE FOODS OF ANIMAL ORIGIN.................. 69

V. THE DISEASES REFERABLE TO FAULTY DIET, OR THE SO-CALLED "DEFICIENCY DISEASES"............. 83

VI. THE NURSING MOTHER AS A FACTOR OF SAFETY IN THE NUTRITION OF THE SUCKLING.................. 116

VII. PRACTICAL CONSIDERATIONS WHICH SHOULD GUIDE IN THE PLANNING OF THE DIET.................. 130

INTRODUCTION TO THE LEGENDS TO THE CHARTS ... 154

BIBLIOGRAPHY................................. 191

INDEX....................................... 197

THE NEWER KNOWLEDGE OF NUTRITION

THE NEWER KNOWLEDGE OF NUTRITION

CHAPTER I

THE BIOLOGICAL METHOD FOR THE ANALYSIS OF A FOOD-STUFF

Our knowledge of nutrition has progressed hand in hand with the development of the science of Chemistry. Chemical science gave us the clue to an understanding of the nature of the food-stuffs and the changes which take place in digestion, as well as an appreciation of some of the secrets of the metabolic processes which take place within the tissues of the body. Chemistry will continue, as time goes on, to aid in extending our knowledge of the finer processes of physiology. Nevertheless, it has been possible for a time to advance very rapidly in the study of nutrition, from the technical as well as from the practical standpoint, by a systematic feeding of simplified diets to animals. The results were interpreted on the observations as to the ability, or failure, of the animals to develop normally, as the diets were modified. Progress has resulted in the past, and will continue in the future to come from the judicious division of labor between the study of food problems by chemical methods, and by animal experimentation. In this brief exposition of the present situation respecting our knowledge of foods and nutrition, it is desirable that the reader should appreciate the viewpoint of the investigator, and should understand the line of reasoning by which the successive steps in the progress of the last few years have been attained. A brief historical account of the steps by which research in this field have been developed will serve this purpose, and at the same time, will illustrate the mental processes of a student engaged in the task of bringing order into a field of scientific inquiry where before there was no clear understanding.

A plant structure, or an animal body is an exceedingly complex mixture of chemical substances, many of which are themselves individually as complicated in their structure as the most complex machine. The first step in the direction of reaching an understanding of the chemistry of the living mass, must involve the separation and study of the structural units of which the tissues are composed. This was, indeed, the field of activity of many organic and physiological chemists during the nineteenth century. The fats and the simpler substances into which they can be converted as in soap making; the starches and the simpler sugars, and the manner in which they are related chemically; the proteins, bodies having the properties of egg white, the casein of milk, hair, etc., yet very closely related in their chemical nature, since they can all be resolved into the same digestion products in the animal body, or in the chemical laboratory, have all been carefully studied and with marked success. These and a long list of a thousand or more relatively simple chemical substances have been discovered, and isolated in a state of purity from plant and animal tissues. They have been studied to determine their special properties, composition and the tests by means of which they may be recognized and identified.

Through a century of patient labor by many able men, an understanding of the number and character of simple structural units into which the tissues of animal or plant can be separated, became realized. Furthermore, certain of these simple bodies could be recognized as intermediate products on their way toward being built up into the most highly organized units of the living tissues; others were shown to be degradation products resulting from the physiological activity of the living tissues of the plant or animal. Through these studies it became established that the body of an animal or the tissues of a plant consists essentially of: proteins, which are peculiar in that they contain about sixteen per cent of the element nitrogen, and are complex in structure; starch-like substances and sugars, into which the starches can be easily converted, and fats and a number of closely related, and, in many respects, similar substances known collectively as lipoids. With these there are always associated in the living tissues more or less

water and a number of mineral salts. Numerous
special varieties of each of these types of substances
became known, and their less obvious characteristics
were described. Certain substances were found to
be special products, found only at certain times and
in certain special localities, and these became regarded in their true light, as of subordinate interest.
Examples of such are the alkaloids, quinine, strich-
nine, etc., the cellulose which serves as skeletal tissue
for the plant but is not necessary for the animal, and
in the same category belong the waste products of
the life processes of the animal body, most of which
are not found in plant substances. Living tissues,
although always associated with numerous substances, the exact importance of which could not
be determined, were found to consist essentially of
the proteins, fats, sugars, mineral salts and water.
These came to be regarded even as early as 1840, as
the essential and never failing constituents of plant
tissues and were regarded as the essential constituents
of an adequate diet for an animal.

The processes of the digestion of food have excited
the wonderment and have occupied the patient
attention of some of the most earnest students of
physiology and biochemistry. The chemistry of the
fats, and the starches and sugars being simpler, or
rather less complex than that of the proteins, came
to be earlier understood in their essential features.
It was not until toward the close of the nineteenth
century that the nature and extent of protein diges-

tion became clearly appreciated. Soon after 1900 the researches of Fischer revealed the great variation in the composition of proteins from different sources.[1] This discovery introduced into nutrition studies the idea of quality in addition to quantity which had heretofore seemed satisfactory to students of nutrition. Most proteins were found to be resolved into eighteen simple digestion products called amino-acids, and it was found that the proportions in which these were present in the protein molecule varied greatly in the proteins from different sources. All or nearly all of these digestion products appear to be indispensable constituents of an adequate diet. All natural foods contain several proteins as the extensive and valuable studies of Osborne have shown,[2] and although there are individual proteins which are entirely lacking in one or more of the essential digestion products of proteins, every natural food appears to contain more or less of each of them. The proteins of any single food-stuff may be regarded as biologically complete, but their biological values differ greatly, depending upon the yield of the several amino-acids which can be obtained from them.

Food Analysis.—Since proteins, carbohydrates, such as starches and sugars, fats and mineral salts came to be regarded as the essential constituents of the normal diet, it early became the principal activity of the investigator of nutrition problems to analyze foods of every sort by chemical methods in order to determine their content of what were supposed to be the only essential food complexes. Pronounced differences were observed in the composition of the many substances which serve as food for man and animals. Meats, milk, eggs, and a few seeds such as the pea and bean are very rich in protein, the cereal grains contain less of this food substance, whereas the tubers and vegetables, especially in the fresh condition, contain but very little. Equally great variations are observable in the water content of foods, and in their yields of fats and carbohydrates. One of the great epochs in the development of the science of nutrition, is that in which Atwater and his associates examined and tabulated in classified form the chemical composition of an extensive list of human foods.[3] Following this, similar data were accumulated in the Agricultural Experiment Stations concerning substances used for animal foods. Up to about 1900 the idea that there was any variation in the quality of the proteins from different sources did not become generally appreciated.

In the light of the revelations in the field of nutrition during the last few years, it seems remarkable that close students of animal nutrition accepted for so long, without proof, the belief that the results of a chemical analysis revealed the dietary values of food-stuffs.

Disease and Diet.—Restricted diets of monotonous character have produced, for centuries, diseases in man in several parts of the world. The only one of these which was at all general in the Western hemisphere was scurvy, a disease which caused much suffering among sailors in the days of the long sailing voyages. It was well understood that the disease was the sequel to the consumption of a faulty diet, composed usually of biscuit and salt meats, and that prompt recovery resulted from the consumption of liberal amounts of fresh vegetables and fruits. Decades passed without any systematic attempt to determine the cause of the peculiar value of this class of foods.

Pellagra was a scourge among the poorest of peasants in parts of Europe for centuries, and its etiology has been referred by many to the poor quality of the simple and monotonous diet. This disease was not observed in America until after 1900. Since then it has been steadily increasing in the Southern States.

Beri-beri is a disease common among the poorest classes of the Orient, who limit their food supply principally to polished rice and fish. It is remarkable that not until the year 1897 was the first fertile suggestion made by Eijkman,[4] as to the nature of the dietary fault which was responsible for the development of this disease.

Man has been sufficiently industrious in most parts of the world to secure for himself a varied diet, derived from the cereal grains and legumes, fruits, roots and tubers, meats and certain leaves, which he found edible. Beginning with the dawn of the era of his most rapid advance toward achievement, he has in many parts of the world been the possessor and protector of flocks and herds, which provided him with clothing, and a constant supply of both meat and milk. The importance of this last item in his food supply we have just now come to really appreciate. It is in order that it may be fully appreciated how great are the differences in the nutritive value of foods of such a composition as to appear alike from the results of chemical analysis that the present account of the investigations of recent years was prepared.

In the year of 1907 the author began the study of nutrition problems at the Wisconsin Experiment Station. An inspection of the literature which related to nutrition at that time disclosed the fact that the diet was supposed to consist essentially of protein, carbohydrates and fats, and a suitable amount of several mineral salts. There were in the literature two papers which were highly suggestive that a new era was about to dawn in this field of research. Henriques and Hansen,[5] believing that gliadin, one of the proteins of wheat, was free from the amino-acid lysine, had made up a diet of purified gliadin, carbohydrate, fats and mineral salts, and had attempted to nourish on this food mixture, animals whose growth was complete. It was reported that rats had been kept in a state of nitrogen equilibrium, and even retention of nitrogen (protein) was reported during an experimental period covering nearly a month. In most of their trials the animals failed steadily from the time they were confined to food of this character.

Willcock and Hopkins [6] had conducted experiments with similar food mixtures, composed of carefully purified food-stuffs in which all the constituents were known. When the protein of the diet consisted solely of zein, from maize, the mice lived but a few days. When to this food the amino-acid tryptophane, which is not obtained on the digestion of zein, was added to the diet, the animals lived distinctly longer than without this addition. All experimental work with such diets indicated that they were unable to support well-being in a young animal during growth over a prolonged period. It was an interest in these results, and a desire to know why such food mixtures, which complied with all the requirements of the chemist and the dietitian, failed to properly nourish an animal that led to the decision that the study of nutrition offered a promising field of activity.

At the Wisconsin Experiment Station there was in progress at that time an experiment which greatly strengthened the author's conviction that the most profitable point of attack for the study of the problems of nutrition, lay in the study of greatly simplified diets so made up that every component should be known. It seemed that, employing such diets, and by the systematic addition of one or more purified substances known to be found in natural foods, or in animal tissues, it should be possible to arrive at the solution of the problem of just what chemical complexes are necessary in the diet of the higher animals.

The above experiment was based upon earlier work by Professor S. M. Babcock, and was suggested by him, and carried out at first by Professors Hart and Humphrey, and later with the coöperation of· Mr. Steenbock and the author.[7] In this experiment the object was to determine whether rations, so made up as to be alike, in so far as could be determined by chemical analysis, but derived each from a single plant, would prove to be of the same value for growth and the maintenance of vigor in cattle.

The ration employed for one group of animals was derived solely from the wheat plant, and consisted of wheat, wheat gluten and wheat straw; for a second group the ration consisted entirely of corn plant products, and included the corn kernel, corn gluten, a by-product of the corn starch industry, and the leaves and stalks of the corn plant (corn stover); the third group derived their ration solely from the oat plant, being fed entirely upon rolled oats and oat straw.   There was a fourth group which it was supposed would serve as controls, which was fed a ration having the same chemical composition, but derived from about equal parts of wheat, corn and oat products.

The animals employed were young heifer calves weighing about 350 pounds, and were as nearly comparable in size and vigor as could be secured.

They were restricted absolutely to the experimental diets, and were well cared for. They were given all the salt (NaCl) they cared to eat, and were allowed to exercise in an open lot free from vegetation. Their behavior during growth, and in performing the functions of reproduction were extremely interesting. All groups ate practically the same amount of feed, and digestion tests showed that there was no difference in the digestibility of the three rations.

It was not until the animals had been confined to their experimental rations for a year or more that distinct differentiation in their appearance was easily observable. The corn fed group were sleek and fine and were evidently in an excellent state of nutrition. In marked contrast stood the wheat fed group. These animals were rough coated and gaunt in appearance and small of girth as compared with those fed the corn plant ration. The weights of the two groups did not differ in a significant degree. The groups fed the oat plant ration and the mixture of the three plants, leaf and seed, stood intermediate between the two lots just described. The assumption that the animals receiving the mixture of products would do better than any of the others, and thus serve as the standard group for controls was not realized. The corn fed animals were at all times in a better state of nutrition than were those receiving the greater variety of food materials.

The reproduction records of these animals are of special interest. The corn fed heifers invariably carried their young the full term, and the young showed remarkable vigor. All were normal in size and were able to stand and suck within an hour after birth as is the rule with vigorous calves. All lived and developed in a normal manner. The young of the wheat fed mothers were the reverse in all respects. All were born three to four weeks too soon, and all were small and weighed on an average forty-six pounds, whereas the young of the corn fed animals weighed 73 to 75 pounds each. This weight is normal for new-born calves. The young were either dead when born or died within a few hours. The young of the mothers which had been grown on the oat plant were almost as large as those from the corn fed mothers, the average weight being 71 pounds. All of them produced their calves about two weeks too soon. One of the four was born dead, two were very weak and died within a day or two after birth, the fourth was weak, but with care it was kept alive. The young of the cows fed the mixture of the three plants were weak in most cases, and one was born dead and one lived but six days. The mothers were kept on their experimental rations, and the following year they repeated in all essential details the reproduction records observed in the first gestation period.

Records were kept of the milk production during the first thirty days of the first lactation period. The average production per day by each individual in the corn-fed lot was 24.03 pounds; for the wheat-fed animals 8.04 pounds, and for the oat-fed animals 19.38 pounds. Those fed the mixture of the three plants produced 19.82 pounds of milk per cow per day during the first thirty days. In the second lactation period the figures for milk production were 28.0; 16.1; 30.1; 21.3 pounds, respectively, per day during the first thirty days.

Through autopsy and analysis of tissues of the young, and analysis of the feces and urines of the animals in the several groups, an elaborate attempt was made to solve the problem of the cause of the marked differentiation of the animals fed these restricted diets. Interesting data were secured which showed marked differences in the character of the fat in the milk of cows from the different lots, and the observation was made that the urines of the wheat fed animals were invariably distinctly acid in reaction, whereas those from the other lots were alkaline or neutral to litmus indicator. It was not possible by any means known to physiological chemistry, to obtain a clue to the cause of the pronounced differences in the physiological well-being of the different lots of cows. This experiment confirmed the author's conviction that the only way in which the problems of nutrition could ever be solved, would be to solve the problem of the successful feeding of the most simplified diets possible. If this were accomplished it would be possible to proceed from the simple to the complex diets employed in practical nutrition, ascertaining the nature of the dietary faults in each of the natural foods, singly, the seed alone, and the leaf alone before attempting to interpret the cause of malnutrition in animals fed the more complex mixtures.

Such an undertaking as that just described, viz., the solution of the problem of why animals do not thrive on a diet of purified protein, starch, sugars, fats and inorganic salts which contained all the elements known to be left, as ash, on the incineration of an animal body, necessitated the employment of small laboratory animals. This was true for several reasons: First, because it is difficult and laborious to prepare isolated and purified food substances in sufficient amounts for the conduct of feeding experiments; second, it is both necessary and desirable to shorten the length of the experiments as much as possible, consistent with obtaining data regarding growth and reproduction, in order that data may accumulate sufficiently fast to make progress reasonably rapid. The domestic rat seemed to be the most suitable animal, and accordingly it was selected. The rat has a gestation period of but 21 days, and the young are ready to wean at the age of 25 days. The female usually produces her first litter of young at the age of about 120 days, and will as a rule have five litters by the time she reaches the age of fourteen months, which age marks the end of her fertility. The span of life of a rat which is well nourished is about 36 months. When such an animal is employed, it is possible to accomplish within a relatively short time, the accumulation of data regarding growth and reproduction which it would take years to secure with domestic animals of large size, long period of gestation and long span of life.

A sufficient number of comparable experiments have now been conducted with several species of animals to make it appear certain that the chemical requirements of one species are the same as that of another among all the higher animals. The requirements with respect to the physical properties of the food vary greatly. The ruminants must have bulky food with the right consistency, whereas the omnivora (man, pig, rat, etc.), cannot, because of the nature of their digestive tracts, consume enough of such foods as leaves and coarse vegetables, to meet their energy requirements.

The early efforts to nourish young rats on diets composed of purified proteins, carbohydrates, fats and mineral salts, confirmed the results of the earlier investigators. The animals lived no longer on such food mixtures, than when allowed to fast. The rations employed were of such a character that the most thorough chemical analysis could reveal no reason why they should not adequately nourish an animal. It seemed obvious that there was something lacking from such mixtures which is indispensable for the nutrition of an animal, and a systematic effort was made during the years that followed to discover the cause of failure of animals to develop on diets of purified and isolated food-stuffs. It was not until 1912 that light began to be shed upon the problem.

The diet which was most in use at that time consisted of purified casein to the extent of about 18 per cent, lactose 20 per cent (supposed to be pure), about 5 per cent of some fat, together with a salt mixture which was made up in imitation of the mineral content of milk, and the remainder of starch to make 100 per cent.[8] This food mixture was supposed to be composed of materials sufficiently pure to comply with the requirements of such work; that is, they were supposed to contain too little of any impurities which would in any way influence the results. With this diet the interesting observation was made *that growth could be secured when the fat in the food mixture was butter fat, whereas no growth could be secured when the butter fat was replaced by lard, olive oil or other vegetable oils.* Egg yolk fats were next tried and were found to induce growth in the same manner as butter fat. It was definitely established that, contrary to the past beliefs, the fats are not all of the same dietary value. Certain fats contain some substance which is not dispensable from the diet, whereas other fats do not contain the dietary essential in question.

The portion of the food mixture other than fat, appeared to contain only substances of known composition, *i. e.*, protein, carbohydrate and inorganic salts, and for a time it appeared that the unknown substance in butter fat was the only element of mystery in the diet. The lactose or milk sugar was carefully examined as to its purity and was judged to be sufficiently pure to be satisfactory for such experimental work, since it was practically free from nitrogen. The tentative conclusion was reached that the essential factors in an adequate diet included one substance or a group of substances which had not been appreciated in the past, and that these, if there should be more than one, were associated with certain fats but not with all.

This observation was in harmony with the published work of Stepp [9] which had appeared in 1909. Stepp observed that grown mice were satisfactorily nourished by a bread which was made with milk, but that early failure and death followed when the animals were fed the same bread which had been previously extracted with alcohol. When the substances extracted from the bread by alcohol were replaced, the bread was again rendered efficient for the maintenance of life and health. He demonstrated in other experiments that the bread could be extracted with ether or with chloroform without removing the substance which was soluble in alcohol, and without which the animals steadily failed. Stepp considered the unknown substance or substances with which he was dealing in his feeding work, as belonging to the not well defined group of substances generally called lipoids. This group includes fats and related substances more complex in character, some of which contain the elements, phosphorous and nitrogen. Stepp was not able to secure with any known lipoid, the effects which resulted from the administration of the alcohol-soluble portion of his milk bread.

A new viewpoint was suggested by F. G. Hopkins of Cambridge, England, in 1912.[10] He had as early as 1906 conducted experiments in the feeding of mixtures of purified protein, carbohydrate, fats and mineral salts and was aware of the fact that neither maintenance of body weight, nor growth could be secured with such diets. He then tried the addition of such amounts of milk as would furnish 4 per cent of the total dry matter of the food mixture and observed that growth could proceed when such milk additions were made. Hopkins suggested the existence of certain unidentified food substances which were supplied by the milk and to these he 'gave the name "accessory" articles of the diet.

Attention has been called to the fact that Eijkman, a student of the disease, beri-beri, made the discovery in 1897 that pigeons fed solely upon polished rice, develop usually within three or four weeks, a state of paralysis which is called polyneuritis, and is analogous to beri-beri in man. He found that when the birds were given the entire rice kernel, or unpolished rice the disease did not develop. It was found, furthermore, that the administration of rice polishings to pigeons suffering from polyneuritis, caused prompt relief of their symptoms. Eijkman's observations attracted little attention until 1911, when

Funk took up the study of beri-beri, and made an elaborate attempt to isolate and study the "curative" substance in rice polishings.[11] Fraser and Stanton had, however, in 1907, employed alcoholic extracts of rice polishings for the relief of experimental polyneuritis.[12] In the work of these investigators the erroneous assumption seems to have prevailed that the process of polishing consists essentially of the removal of the outer covering, or bran layer of the rice kernel. As a matter of fact the rice germ is in a very exposed position, and is easily rubbed off during the process of polishing. As was later shown by McCollum and Davis, for the wheat kernel, the germ is a very different thing from the seed from the dietary standpoint.[13] The reason for this will be made clear later.

The studies of Eijkman, Hopkins, Fraser and Stanton and Funk, referred to above, clearly suggested that there was required in the diet something other than protein, carbohydrate, fats and inorganic salts. When McCollum and Davis succeeded in securing growth in young rats fed upon a mixture of "purified" food-stuffs, when the mixture contained butter fat, but no growth when vegetable fats or the body fats of animals were substituted, it appeared to them that the only element of mystery in the diet was that associated with certain fats. This could not at first be harmonized with the observation of Funk, namely, that butter fat had no favorable influence on pigeons which were suffering from experimental beri-beri.[14]   His studies seemed to indicate that there is necessary in the normal diet at least one other substance, the absence of which brought on the attack of polyneuritis. Later experiments by McCollum and Davis cleared up the problem, but not without a considerable amount of experimenting and delay.

McCollum and Davis arrived at the conclusion that aside from the long recognized constituents of the normal diet, there is some unknown substance in butter fat which must likewise be furnished in the food, and began a systematic investigation of the problem of why a young animal cannot grow when restricted to a single grain such as wheat, maize (corn), oats, peas, beans, etc. They had tried many times to limit young rats to whole wheat, or other grain as their sole food, and had. found that they not only failed to grow, but would not live many weeks. Chemical analysis shows the cereal grains to contain all the essential food substances, for which we know how to analyze, viz: proteins, starch, sugar, fats and all the mineral salts which occur in the body of an animal.

It was reasoned that, since all the dietary essentials, except possibly the one which is not present in vegetable fats, are certainly present in the wheat kernel, the faults in the latter must depend upon a lack of the unknown substance contained in butter fat, or on the quality of some one or more of the well recognized constituents of the diet. It seemed possible to discover by means of a systematic series of feeding experiments in which the quality of the seed should be improved with respect to one dietary factor at a time, which factor was interfering with growth. Accordingly they fed wheat in the following combinations, and with the results noted:

(1) Wheat alone......................no growth, short life.
(2) Wheat plus purified protein.........no growth, short life.
(3) Wheat plus a salt mixture which gave it a mineral content
    similar to that of milk.............very little growth.
(4) Wheat plus a growth promoting fat (butter-fat)
                                       no growth.

From these results it seemed apparent that either their working hypothesis regarding the factors which are necessary in an adequate diet, must be wrong, or there must be more than a single dietary factor of poor quality, and jointly responsible for the poor nutrition of the animals. In order to test this theory they carried out another series of feeding experiments, in which wheat was fed, supplemented with two purified food additions.

(5) Wheat plus protein, plus the salt mixture..........Good
                                growth for a time.   Few
                                or no young.   Short life.
(6) Wheat plus protein, plus a growth-promoting fat (butter-
    fat).......................No growth.   Short life.
(7) Wheat plus the salt mixture, plus the growth-promoting fat,
    (butter-fat)............Fair growth for a time.   Few
                                or no young.   Short life.

The behavior of the animals fed wheat with two purified food additions was highly suggestive that there are three dietary factors of poor quality in the wheat kernel. This was demonstrated to be true by a feeding trial in which wheat was fed with three purified food additions:

(8) Wheat plus protein, plus the salt mixture, plus a growth-promoting fat (butter-fat) ....Good growth, normal number of young, good success in rearing young; life approximately the normal span.

McCollum and Davis were, in 1912, more than ever convinced that the only element of mystery in the normal diet was the unidentified substance in butter fat, for with the improvement of three dietary factors wheat became a satisfactory food for the nutrition of an animal during growth and for the support of all the functions of reproduction and rearing of young.

This series of experiments brought to light two new viewpoints in animal nutrition, one of which was, *that the inorganic content of the wheat kernel, although it furnishes all the necessary elements, does not contain enough of certain of these to meet the requirements of a young animal during the growing period.* It is true that some years earlier Henry,[15] had called attention to the deficiency of the corn kernel in ash constituents, and had in some of his experiments added wood ashes to the diet, with noticeable improvement in the well-being of the animals. The fact that seeds such as wheat fail to supply enough of any of the essential inorganic elements was not generally appreciated and was given but little attention in works on nutrition. Later, work by McCollum and Simmonds, demonstrated that the deficiency in mineral elements in wheat and other seeds is limited to three elements, calcim, sodium and chlorine.

A second new viewpoint brought out by these experiments was the fact that the wheat kernel is indeed too poor in its content of the unidentified substance which butter fat contains, to satisfactorily nourish an animal over a long period of time.

It has already been mentioned that the studies of Kossel, Fischer and of Osborne, had made it clear that there should exist very pronounced differences in the value of the proteins from different sources. The proteins were prepared in a state of relative purity and were digested in the laboratory by means of acids, and were analyzed by the methods of Fischer and of Kossel. Certain of the eighteen digestion products, the amino-acids, were determined quantitatively so far as the methods would permit. Although the methods were never perfected so as to give results which were approximately quantitative, except in the case of less than a third of the amino-acids which were known to be formed in the digestion of proteins, it was shown in the case of these few that there were very great variations in the proportions among them in the mixture obtained from proteins from different sources. Thus the proteins of the muscle tissues of several species of animals were shown to yield between 12 and 14 per cent of glutamic acid, one of the digestion products obtained from practically all proteins. The same amino-acid. is present in the two principal proteins of the wheat kernel to the extent of about 40 per cent of the total protein. These two proteins together make about 85 per cent of the total protein of the wheat kernel. Other equally great differences were shown to exist in the composition of proteins of our common food-stuffs and those of the tissue proteins which are formed during growth.

A good illustration of the problems which the animal meets in its protein nutrition, may be had by comparing the digestion products of the protein molecule to the letters of the alphabet. The proteins of the food and of the tissues are made up of the same letters arranged in different orders and present in different proportions. In growth the animal takes as food, proteins which are very unlike those of its tissues, digests these into the simple complexes, the amino-acids, and then, after absorbing these, puts together the fragments in new order, and in new proportions to form the tissue proteins.

If the muscle tissue of an animal be likened to a block of printer's type so arranged as to print the rhyme beginning "Jack Spratt, who could eat no fat, and his wife could eat no lean," the proteins of which the muscle consists are represented by the individual words, and the digestion products of the proteins by the letters of which the words consist. Now if the animal could take in its food proteins which correspond to a block of type which would print the jingle beginning: "Peter Piper picked a peck of pickled peppers," it is easy to understand that when the proteins of the food are resolved to their constituent letters, and an effort made to form the body proteins of the new and different type from the letters supplied by the food, the transformation cannot be made. In setting up the first line, "Jack Spratt could eat no fat and his wife could eat no lean," we need four of the letter t, but the food proteins contain but one. The first line of the Jack Spratt rhyme, which represents the muscle proteins, requires but one letter p, whereas the food proteins represented by the Peter Piper rhyme yield nine in the first line. The first line of the Jack Spratt rhyme contains the letters j and n, whereas the Peter Piper rhyme contains none, so that even with the entire stanza:

Peter Piper picked a peck of pickled peppers
If Peter Piper picked a peck of pickled peppers,
Where's the peck of pickled peppers,
That Peter Piper picked?

it is not possible to reproduce even the first line of the Jack Spratt rhyme, and in order that growth might become possible, it would be necessary to take proteins of another character, which would supply the missing letters.

Such a comparison between food proteins and tissue proteins gives a good illustration of the kind of problem which the animal meets in its protein nutrition. The most conspicuous protein of the corn kernel (zein) is wholly lacking in three of the amino-acids or digestion products which are obtainable from most tissue proteins. In accord with what we should expect on theoretical grounds, this protein is, when taken as the sole source of amino-acids, not capable of supporting growth, or of maintaining an animal in body weight. This illustration shows how we may have excellent, good or poor food proteins for the formation of body proteins in growth.

The investigations described above, the object of which was to find the cause of the failure of an animal to grow when restricted to wheat as its sole source of nutriment, were carried out in 1912, the year following the publication of the first work by Funk on polyneuritis. In the same year Hopkins called attention to the remarkable effects produced by the addition of small amounts of milk to diets composed of purified food-stuffs. The "vitamine" hypothesis had just been formulated by Funk.[16] McCollum and Davis were, therefore, aware of the relation of a diet of polished rice to experimental beri-beri. They believed, in the light of their experiences with the diet of purified protein, carbohydrate, fats and inorganic salts, which, they observed, was capable of inducing growth when certain fats were supplied, but not when others were substituted, and the further fact that wheat could be supplemented by purified protein, a growth-promoting fat, and a suitable salt mixture, i. e. with food-stuffs of known character, that there was but a single unidentified substance necessary in the diet. They decided to next apply to polished rice the same procedure which had shown so clearly the nature of the dietary deficiencies of wheat. Rice, they reasoned, could be nothing less than a mixture of proteins, starch, traces of fat, and a mixture of inorganic salts, similar to that contained in wheat, but smaller in amount. It should, therefore, be supplemented with a suitable salt mixture, a purified protein, and a growth-promoting fat, so as to induce growth and maintain animals for a long time in a state of health. This seemed to be a necessary conclusion, since they had secured growth and well-being in animals fed strictly upon a mixture of purified protein (casein), starch, milk-sugar, butter fat and a mixture of inorganic salts of suitable composition.

It was a great surprise to McCollum and Davis to find that polished rice, even when supplemented with the purified protein, casein, butter fat and a salt mixture properly constituted, failed utterly to induce any growth in young rats.[17]   Not only did they fail to grow, but in the course of a few weeks they developed in some cases a state of paralysis which was suggestive of polyneuritis. Here was an apparent contradiction. The polished rice could be nothing less than a mixture of protein, carbohydrate and salts. The only difference between this and the mixture of supposedly purified food-stuffs with which they had achieved success was in the 20 per cent of milk sugar which the latter contained. It was, therefore, decided to repeat the experiments with the latter mixture, with the milk sugar replaced by starch. It was found that this change in the composition of the food mixture made the difference between success and failure. No growth could be secured when the milk sugar was omitted. Later experiments showed that if milk sugar was sufficiently purified by repeated crystallization it was no longer effective in inducing growth when added to the purified food mixture; whereas the water from which the sugar had been crystallized would, when evaporated upon the food mixture, render it capable of inducing growth. This made it evident that there is indeed a second dietary essential, of which an animal needs but a very small amount, but which is absolutely necessary for both growth in the young and the maintenance of health in the adult.

Further experiments were then conducted to find whether this unidentified substance which was being added accidentally as an impurity in the milk sugar, was the same as the substance which Fraser and Stanton and Funk were dealing with in their studies of beri-beri. It was found that pigeons which had developed beri-beri as the result of being fed exclusively upon polished rice, could be temporarily "cured" with any preparation which would, when added to the diet of purified food-stuffs, containing a growth-promoting fat, cause animals to grow.

Following the method introduced by Fraser and Stanton, McCollum and Davis,[18] next employed alcoholic extracts of various natural foods, adding the alcohol soluble matter to the standard mixture of purified protein (casein), starch (dextrinized), salts and butter fat, and soon became convinced that the substance which relieves the condition of polyneuritis in pigeons was always present in the preparations which render the purified food mixture capable of promoting growth. They finally adopted an alcoholic extract of wheat germ as a source of this dietary factor in their investigations. Funk and his co-workers had previously shown that the curative substance is present in many natural foods.[16] Repeated trials showed that the inclusion of the alcoholic extract of wheat germ or of other food, was not sufficient to induce growth *unless the butter fat was likewise added to the purified food mixture. Both the growth-promoting fat and the trace of unidentified substance in the alcoholic extract of wheat germ are necessary for the promotion of growth or the preservation of health.*

It has been pointed out that Funk, in his examination of the various natural foods for the purpose of

determining the distribution of the antineuritic substance (substance which relieves polyneuritis) found
butter fat ineffective. This was later confirmed by
McCollum and Kennedy.[19]

Through the "vitamine" hypothesis, Funk attempted to account for the diseases beri-beri, scurvy,
pellagra and rickets, as being each due to the lack
of a specific chemical substance, a "vitamine," in
the diet.[16] This was a very logical conclusion from
the data available to Funk. Scurvy, it had long
been known is relieved in a very spectacular manner
by the inclusion of fresh vegetables or orange juice
in the diet, and there was no doubt that the disease
developed as the result of a diet of poor quality. On
first consideration it seemed very reasonable to
assume that there is an "antiscorbutic vitamine"
in certain fruits and vegetables.

Pellagra has long been suspected of being due to
faulty diet, although the exact manner in which the
diet is unsatisfactory remained obscure. It was
generally appreciated by clinicians that a change to
a highly nutritious diet in which milk and eggs were
conspicuous was the best prophylactic measure for
the treatment of the disease, and that without dietary measures, all remedies fail. It was not surprising that Funk should have regarded pellagra as one
of the "deficiency" diseases, due to lack of a "vitamine" in the diet. As will be shown later (Chapter V)
there has since been secured much experimental evidence in support of the view that scurvy and pellagra

do not arise from deficiency in the diet of specific chemical substances in the sense in which Funk suggested. This seems to be true also of rickets.

In view of the considerations just mentioned relative to the cause of scurvy and pellagra, and the convincing evidence that beri-beri is actually caused by specific starvation for a substance, "vitamine," as Funk suggested, McCollum and Davis formulated in the following way, their working hypothesis as to what constitutes an adequate diet. The diet must contain, in addition to the long recognized dietary factors, viz: protein, a source of energy in the form of proteins, carbohydrates and fats; a suitable supply of certain inorganic salts, two as yet unidentified substances or groups of substances.[18] One of these is associated with certain fats, and is especially abundant in butter fat, egg yolk fats and the fats of the glandular organs such as the liver and kidney, but is not found in any fats or oils of vegetable origin. The second substance or group of substances of chemically unidentified nature, is never associated with fats or oils of either animal or vegetable origin. It is widely distributed in natural foods, and can be isolated in a concentrated, but not in a pure form, from natural food-stuffs by extraction of the latter with either water or alcohol. This water or alcoholic extract always contains the substance which cures polyneuritis. At the time it seemed possible that it also contained several other "vitamines," protective against the other diseases mentioned. The former substance or group of substances, which is associated with certain fats is not "curative" for any of the list of diseases which Funk designated as "vitamine" deficiency diseases. Indeed, butter fat, which is the food containing one of the indispensable substances in greatest abundance, was stated by Funk to contain no "vitamine.'" [14]

Nomenclature of the Unidentified Dietary Essentials.—The ending *amine* has a definite and specific meaning in organic chemistry, and applies only to substances containing the element nitrogen. Since butter fat, which is very rich in one of the dietary essentials in question is practically, if not entirely, free from nitrogen, it seems almost certain that the physiologically indispensable substance which it contains is free from nitrogen, and could not with propriety be designated by any name ending in *amine*. For this reason, and because it is possible to divide the unidentified constituents of the normal diet into two classes on the basis of their solubility, McCollum and Kennedy [19] proposed the terms fat-soluble A and water-soluble B to designate them. The former prevents the development of a pathological condition of the eyes,[20] the latter prevents the development of beri-beri. As will be shown later, there is much evidence for and none against the view that what we designate by each of these terms is in reality but a single physiologically indispensable substance and not a group of substances. This necessitates the further assumption that certain of the diseases of dietary origin, which Funk held to be due to "vi-tamine" starvation, are in reality due to other causes. This view will be supported by further evidence later. Indeed it is not possible to longer regard scurvy as a "vitamine" deficiency disease.

The "vitamine" hypothesis of Funk was extremely attractive and seemed to account for the etiology of several diseases in a most satisfactory way. It seemed to rest upon sound observations, but in reality it rested only upon suggestive chemical evidence. It failed to stand the test of a systematic investigation of all the more important natural food-stuffs, by the biological method which was described in its essential features in illustrating the nature of the dietary deficiencies of the wheat kernel.

CHAPTER II

EXPERIMENTAL SCURVY AND THE DIETARY PROPERTIES
OF VEGETABLES

McCollum, Simmonds and Pitz [1] sought to test the validity of the "vitamine" hypothesis in its relation to scurvy, by an indirect method. The next logical step in the investigation of the possible number of dietary essentials of unknown chemical nature which occur in the growth-promoting fats (fat-soluble A), and in the preparations which are never associated with fats (water-soluble B), seemed to be to study the oat kernel. There seemed much reason to believe that this seed would prove to be unique among the ordinary seeds in its dietary properties. Theobald Smith [2] had, in 1895, called attention to the fact that a diet of oats would cause in guinea pigs the development of a condition suggestive of scurvy. In 1909 Holst and his co-workers in Sweden [3] described numerous experiments involving the production and relief of experimental scurvy in the guinea pig. Holst observed that when this animal is restricted to a diet of oats it rarely fails to develop scurvy within a few weeks. The disease which is so produced is strikingly suggestive of scurvy in man. There is pronounced swelling of the knee and elbow joints, with rupture of the capillaries at these sites,

34

and there is also a spongy and hemorrhagic condition of the gums.

Holst stated that the disease was due to a deficiency of the oat kernel in an antiscorbutic substance, which is relatively unstable when manipulated in the laboratory. Milk was stated to be efficient for the cure of the disease induced by an oat diet, provided it was raw or had not been heated to very high temperatures. Milk which had been heated to 90° C. for ten minutes was said to be still effective, but boiled milk failed to induce a cure. Raw cabbage was stated to be highly efficient as a remedy against the disease in the guinea pig, whereas cooked or dried cabbage had lost most of its antiscorbutic property.

In view of these observations, it seemed that, if it were true that scurvy is as Funk and Holst believed, a disease resulting from "vitamine" deficiency, the oat kernel should prove to be a natural food-stuff which lacked the antiscorbutic "vitamine" but contained the anti-beri-beri, and perhaps, also, the anti-pellagra and other "vitamines." McCollum, Simmonds and Pitz[1] submitted the oat kernel to the systematic procedure of the biological method of analysis, feeding it as the sole source of nutriment, and also with single and multiple additions of purified food substances, employing the rat as the experimental animal. (This showed that the oat kernel (rolled oats) can be supplemented by the addition of a salt mixture of appropriate composition, a growth-promoting fat, and the purified protein gelatin, so as to induce growth at the maximum rate in young rats from weaning time to the full adult size, and supported the production of a few young. When any one of these additions is omitted, the animals fail to develop. 〉

The oat kernel, therefore, contains all the dietary essentials in the *water-soluble group* (provided there is more than one such substance). Like wheat it lacks a sufficient amount of the fat-soluble A to support normal nutrition. It was impossible to harmonize the results described by Holst in the production of experimental scurvy in the guinea pig with those of McCollum, Simmonds and Pitz, in which the rat served as the experimental animal, without making assumptions which would greatly complicate the whole subject of nutrition investigations. There were serious discrepancies in the experimental data from different sources. Holst's studies pointed to the existence in the normal diet of a substance or substances of unknown character, which were easily destroyed by heat or by dessication, and which act as protective agents against scurvy in the guinea pig, and appeared to demonstrate that the supposed antiscorbutic substance or substances were absent from the oat kernel. The studies with the rat demonstrated beyond controversy, that at least for the rat, the oat kernel is deficient as a food only as respects the factors, inorganic salts, fat-soluble A, and in a lesser degree in the quality of its protein. When these factors are corrected, the oat kernel becomes a complete food for this species.

Scurvy has been produced experimentally by faulty diet in the guinea pig, and is not known to occur in any species other than man and the guinea pig. If the explanation of Holst and of Funk is correct that scurvy is the result of the lack of a specific substance in the diet, it becomes necessary to make the further assumption that man and the guinea pig require this substance, since both suffer from the disease, whereas other species, as the rat, do not require this complex as a dietary component. The only alternative is to conclude that scurvy is in realty not a "deficiency" disease in the sense in which Funk and Holst employed the term. That there is actually no such unstable "antiscorbutic substance" or "antiscorbutic vitamine" as postulated by Holst and Funk, has been demonstrated by the studies of McCollum and Pitz.[4] The proof of this is given in Chapter V. In the same chapter will be discussed the other so-called "vitamine" deficiency diseases, pellagra and rickets, and the character of the diets which play a part in their etiology. The data available supports the view that among the list of so-called "deficiency" diseases, beri-beri, scurvy, pellagra and rickets, only the first is due to the lack of a specific protective substance, Funk's "vitamine," or water-soluble B in the diet. The others are at least in some degree the result of faulty diets, but not in the sense in which Funk and Holst employed the term "deficiency." McCollum and Simmonds have pointed out, however, that in the pathological condition of the eyes, known as xerophthalmia, of dietary origin mentioned above, we have a second deficiency disease, analogous to beri-beri.[5] All the facts at present available point, therefore, to the belief that what McCollum and his co-workers term water-soluble B, is in reality but a single physiologically indispensable substance.[6] There is no evidence in support of the view that the term fat-soluble A need be considered as applying to more than a single chemical substance. Xeropthalmia of dietary origin will be described later (Chapter V).

Similarity of the Seeds from the Dietary Standpoint. —By the application of the biological method of analysis of a food-stuff to each of the more important seeds employed in the nutrition of man and animals, the fact was brought to light that they all resemble each other very closely in their dietary properties. The list of seeds examined included,— wheat,[7] corn,[8] rice,[17] rolled oats, rye,[9] barley,[9] kaffir corn,[9] millet seed,[10] flaxseed,[10] pea[10] and both the navy[11] and the soy bean.[9] (These all contain proteins which are of distinctly lower biological value for growth than are the proteins of milk; they all are too poor in the same three inorganic elements, calcium, sodium and chlorine. All are, with the exception of millet seed, below the optimum in their content of the dietary factor, fat-soluble A. These three diet-

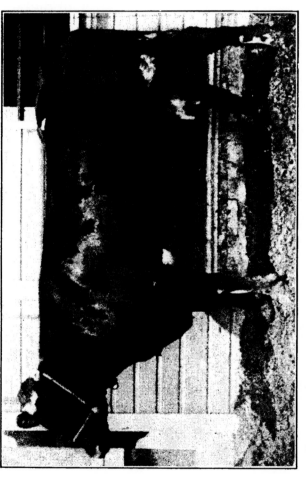

FIG. 1.—Photograph of a cow which grew up on a ration derived solely from the corn plant. The seed, straw and leaf of the plant were all included in the food mixture. Her nutrition was excellent, as shown by her appearance, the vigor of her offspring and her ability to produce an abundance of milk. Figure 2 shows a photograph of her calf, taken soon after it was born. Rations consisting of the entire plant may be highly satisfactory. The seed of the plant is never in itself a complete food.

ary factors must be improved before any one of these seeds becomes complete from the dietary standpoint. The seeds are, therefore, to be classed together as regards their food values. ⌡

Since the seeds have the same faults from the dietary standpoint, it is to be expected that when fed in mixtures they should not supplement each other except as regards the protein moiety. It would hardly be expected that the proteins of two or more kinds of seeds should be deficient in the same amino-acids, and in the same degree, and feeding trials have shown that mixtures of seeds furnish better protein values for growth than do the single seeds when fed alone, properly supplemented with respect to all other factors. (From the similarity of the inorganic content of all seeds, and their low content of the fat-soluble A, it should be necessary to supplement any mixture of seeds with respect to both these factors before good nutrition can be secured. Experimental trial shows this to be the case. *It is not, therefore, possible to secure appreciable growth in young animals fed exclusively upon seed products as the sole source of nutriment.* ⌡

Casual observation teaches us that such animals as the ox, horse, sheep and goat can grow and live for years in a vigorous condition on diets derived entirely from vegetable sources. After having unsuccessfully attempted numerous times to induce growth in animals fed strictly upon seed mixtures, the thought naturally arose that there must be some special properties in the leaves of the plant which cause them to make good the dietary deficiencies of the seeds. A careful inquiry in every possible direction failed to discover any animal which in its natural state limits its diet strictly to seeds. Birds all appear to vary their diet of seeds with insects and worms, and most birds eat to some extent of fruits and certain tender leaves. All birds probably eat a considerable amount of mineral substance in the form of particles which they deliberately swallow, and they secure in their natural state more or less of all of the essential mineral elements in the drinking water which has permeated the ground. These supplemental sources of certain food substances, which one is at first inclined to overlook, or if considered, to regard as of an accessory nature, and therefore, if "accessory," dispensable, are in reality of such importance, that it is not too much to say that the preservation of the species might turn upon the opportunity or lack of opportunity to secure these substances.

Among the omnivora, the author has been unable to discover any species which subsists entirely upon seeds. The hog is a typical omniverous feeder, but it is well known to animal husbandrymen that there are but two successful methods of pork production, one of which is to feed growing pigs on grain while they have access to a good pasture; the other is to feed them milk, skim milk, or butter-milk, along with a grain mixture. Ignorance of this fact has re-

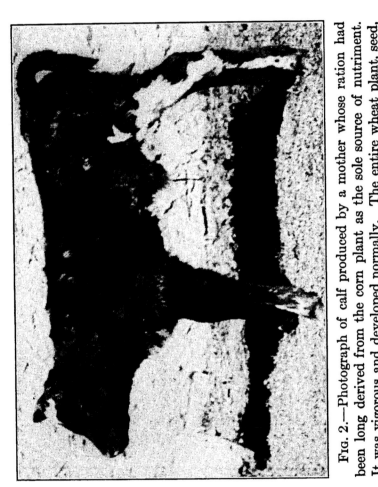

FIG. 2.—Photograph of calf produced by a mother whose ration had been long derived from the corn plant as the sole source of nutriment. It was vigorous and developed normally. The entire wheat plant, seed, leaf and stem make a diet which can support growth, but not good nutrition. The corn kernel alone does not induce growth.

sulted in enormous economic loss to farmers who have attempted to keep growing pigs in a dry lot and feed them cereal grains and by-products derived from these, as the sole source of nutriment. Little growth can be secured under these circumstances, and the reason becomes clear from what has been said above concerning the nature of the dietary deficiencies of the seeds and the similarity of the seeds from the dietary standpoint.*

It was a great surprise to McCollum, Simmonds and Pitz [12] to find that appropriate mixtures of leaf and seed make fairly satisfactory food mixtures for the support of growth, whereas, as has been stated, they were unable to secure any appreciable growth in animals fed exclusively on seeds and seed products, the drinking water supplied being distilled and therefore salt free. The first leaf which was studied was that of the alfalfa plant, for the reason that the ground, immature alfalfa plant is extensively marketed as a supplementary feed for pigs, and through the courtesy of the Peters Milling Company of Omaha, Nebraska a product "alfalfa flour" was made available in a convenient form. This consists

---

* It is not to be understood from this that it is intended to imply that no increase in body weight can be secured in hogs when they are confined strictly to grain mixtures. They may indeed become very fat, and therefore apparently *grow* for a time on such foods as corn alone. Even under farm conditions, where they are able to secure a supplementary mineral supply through the water they drink and through the consumption of soil with the grain, there is little growth in the sense that the muscle and organ tissues increase in volume.

of the dry, immature leaf of the plant ground to a very fine powder of a bright green color.

A series of diets consisting of seed, 60 per cent, and of alfalfa leaf flour, 40 per cent, were first fed to growing rats. The seeds employed, included wheat, corn, rolled oat, rye, millet seed, kaffir corn, pea and bean. The .degree of success in inducing growth with most of these simple mixtures of one seed with the alfalfa leaf is much greater than can ever be secured with even such complex mixtures of seeds as corn, wheat, oat, hemp seed and millet seed in equal proportions. The latter mixture can support a fair amount of growth when its inorganic deficiencies are made good, but without mineral additions almost no growth can be secured. Chart 6 shows typical growth curves which give an accurate idea of the relative values for growth of several combinations of the alfalfa leaf with seeds. Among the seeds with which studies have been made, the oat is best supplemented by the alfalfa leaf. A simple mixture of rolled oats, 60 per cent, and alfalfa leaf, 40 per cent, induces nearly normal growth to the adult size in the rat and induces a fair amount of reproduction and rearing of young. However, the animals fall considerably below the maximum performance in both these respects.

An examination of other leaves of plants showed that the latter can in a general way be classed together as food-stuffs of similar character, since they resemble each other more or less closely, just as the

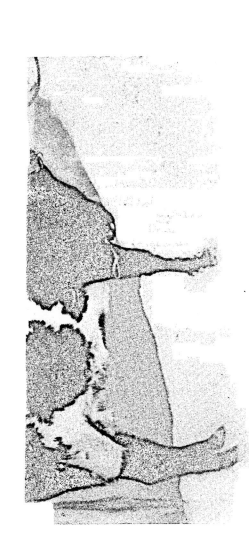

FIG. 3.—This cow was the same age as that shown in Figure 1. She derived her ration entirely from the wheat plant during the last two-thirds of her growing period. This ration ... when ... to ... analysis, showed ... exactly the same composition as that fed to the cow in Figure 1. Note the poor nutritive ... ... of the wheat-fed cow. It has not been ... to prepare a ration solely from wheat products, which will induce good nutrition in animals. Figure 4 shows the typical appearance of the ... fed by cows fed upon a ration properly "...," but derived entirely from the wheat plant, and containing the seed, stem and leaf.

seeds all resemble each other in their dietary properties. The leaf proves to be a very different thing
from the seed from the dietary standpoint. The dry
leaf usually contains from three to five times as
much total ash constituents as does the seed, and
is always especially rich in just those elements in
which the seed is poorest, viz., calcium, sodium and
chlorine. It follows, therefore, that the leaf supplements the inorganic deficiencies of the seed. The
leaf, in most cases, contains much more of the dietary
essential, fat-soluble A, than is found in any seed,
so that combinations of leaf and seed prove more
satisfactory for the nutrition of an animal than do
mixtures of seeds alone. The leaf contains protein
and amino-acids which result from digestion of proteins as does the seed. The amount varies from 8
per cent of protein (nitrogen $\times$ 6.25) in such fleshy
leaves as the cabbage, after drying, to more than
15 per cent in the dry alfalfa or clover leaf. The
seeds vary in their content of protein from about 10
to 25 per cent. The leaf proteins appear, from
the data available, to supplement and enhance in
some degree the value of the seed proteins with which
they are combined. The leaf supplements, therefore,
all the nutritive deficiencies of the seed, but not
necessarily in a highly satisfactory manner.

It is interesting to reflect upon the reasons why
the leaf of the plant should show such decided differences in its nutritive properties as contrasted
with the seed. A consideration of the difference in

function of the two gives the clue to the cause. The seed consists of a germ, which forms in most cases but a very small part of the entire seed, together with a relatively large endosperm. The germ consists of living cells, which respire and are capable of multiplication (germination) when the conditions are favorable. In the wheat kernel the germ constitutes about 5 per cent of the entire seed. The endosperm, on the other hand, consists largely of reserve food materials such as protein, starch, sugars, fats and mineral salts. It is not living matter, and contains few cellular elements. The endosperm is, therefore, in most respects comparable to a mixture of purified food-stuffs. There is, as experiments have abundantly demonstrated, relatively little of the dietary factor, water-soluble B, in the endosperm, and relatively much in the germ or embryo. The same is true for the second unidentified dietary factor fat-soluble A. This is practically absent from the endosperm, but is fairly abundant in the germ. Since the latter represents so small a portion of the entire seed, the seed itself is too poor in this substance, in nearly all cases, to supply the needs of a growing animal.

The leaf of the plant, on the other hand, is very rich in cells, and in most cases contains but little reserve food material. It is the laboratory of the plant. Chlorophyll, its green pigment, enables it to make use of the energy of the sunlight, and from the carbonic acid gas which it absorbs from the air,

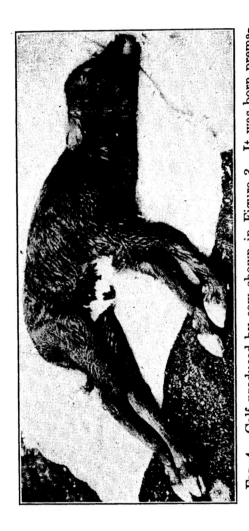

Fig. 4.—Calf produced by cow shown in Figure 3. It was born prematurely, weighed but little more than half as much as calves normally do at birth, and was dead when born. The importance of the source of the food supply, both for the nutrition of mother and the unborn young is strikingly illustrated by these animals. (Figures 1 to 4 are from Research Bulletin 17 of the Wisconsin Experiment Station.)

together with water and mineral salts, which it absorbs from the soil through its roots, it builds up proteins, starch, sugars and fats, which are used for the growth of new plant tissue, or for storage in the seed, tuber or other storage organs. The surfaces of the leaf are a mosaic of living cells. They contain all the chemical complexes which are necessary for the nutrition of the animal cells, and are qualitatively complete foods.

The quality of the leaf from the dietary standpoint may vary to a considerable extent. Some leaves are thin cellular structures, which dry easily in the sun when separated from the plant. In others, as the cabbage, the leaf is in some degree modified as a storage organ, and contains a considerable amount of sugars. The cabbage leaf likewise contains more than the ordinary amount of cellulose, which is its skeletal tissue. Its dietary properties are modified by these peculiarities in that the cellular elements are diluted by the more inert tissues and reserve food substances in the leaf. The freer a leaf is from the function of a storage tissue, the more intensified will be its leaf properties as a food. The fleshy leaves tend to have in some degree the dietary properties of the seed, and stand intermediate between the leaves, which are thin, and dry easily, and the seed in this respect.

The Tubers.—After the seeds, the tubers of certain plants constitute one of the most important classes of energy-yielding foods. The potato and

sweet potato are by far the most important representatives of this group in Europe and the Amer-
icas, but several other kinds of tubers are widely
used as human food in the Orient. An examination
of the potato has been recently made, which reveals
the special dietary properties of this tuber to be just
what we should expect from its function as a storage
organ for reserve food in the plant. The functions
of the potato are twofold, viz., to reproduce the
plant in the following generation, and to furnish
a food supply for the young potato plantlet while
it is developing root and leaf systems which make
it independent of the food stored in the old tuber.
The "eyes" of the potato represent groups of cells
which are analogous to the germ of the seed. These
are the points at which the potato sprouts when the
conditions are appropriate. There is underneath
the skin of the potato a layer of cells which are alive
and respiring during the life of the tuber, but the
interior of the potato consists almost entirely of
water, starch, protein, and to some extent of mineral
salts. The cellular structures in the interior are
gorged with starch, etc., and this portion is therefore
analogous in its dietary properties with the endosperm of the seed. Both are comparable to a mixture
of purified protein, carbohydrate, and salts, which,
as we have previously seen, is not capable of supporting life. This portion, like the portion of the rice
kernel, which remains after polishing, is almost
lacking in both the chemically unidentified dietary

essentials, fat-soluble A and water-soluble B, and accordingly cannot support life even though it may have an appropriate chemical composition as shown by analysis. The potato is to be classed with the seeds in its dietary properties, because it consists largely of reserve food materials and relatively little of cellular elements. The results available indicate that if the potato is steamed and the thin paperlike skin removed without the loss of the cellular layer which lies just underneath, it will contain relatively more of the fat-soluble A, a lack of which leads to the development of the peculiar eye conditions previously described, than do the cereal grains. Although it has not been subjected to experimental test, it would seem that a potato which is pared in the ordinary way and the paring discarded, is changed in its dietary properties in much the same way as is the rice kernel during the polishing process. In the latter, the germ and the bran layer are both rubbed off, leaving the endosperm without the small quota of cellular elements which it possessed in its natural state, and is correspondingly changed in its food value (see legend to Chart 3). The protein of the potato is not quite so valuable for growth as that of the cereal grains when fed as the sole source of this dietary factor.[9]

There have been a number of experiments of short duration which gave results which indicate that in the human subject the nitrogen of the potato is of extraordinary value for replacing that lost through daily metabolism in the adult. McCollum, Simmonds and Parsons, have tested this question by comparing with the protein of the cereal grains the value of the nitrogen of the potato when this tuber was supplemented in such a manner as to make good all of its deficiencies except protein. The experiments involved growth tests in the young rat. The results show conclusively that potato nitrogen falls considerably below the value for growth possessed by the individual cereal grains, when each of. these serves as the sole supply of the digestion products of protein.

The Roots Employed as Food.— The same reasoning applies to the root crops as to the potato, with respect to the relation between dietary properties and biological function. The roots which we employ as food are those which are highly modified as storage organs, and resemble the potato in containing a very high water and starch content, and but very little protein. Like the potato, there is a cellular layer at the periphery, and the interior is loaded with reserve food-stuffs. Appropriate feeding tests have shown that the properties of the beet resemble those of the seed and the tuber, rather than those of the leaf.[9] The fleshy roots and the potato and the sweet potato have an inorganic content which resembles that of the seed in a general way, so that an inspection of the analytical data relating to the composition of the ash of the seeds, tubers and roots, gave no promise that the combination in diets of seeds with either of the latter classes of food-stuffs would correct the inorganic deficiencies of the former. Feeding experiments in which a seed and a tuber were combined, and so supplemented with purified protein, and fat-soluble A (in butter-fat), that all the deficiencies of the mixture, except the inorganic, were made good, have shown that in the combinations of each of the more important seeds with the potato, the resulting mineral supply, which is derived solely from the natural foods themselves, is not of a character suitable for the support of growth.[9] The content of the elements, calcium, sodium and chlorine must be augumented by greater amounts before such food mixtures are complete with respect to their mineral content. No studies have as yet been made to determine the biological value of the nitrogen of the tubers other than the potato, and none at all of the edible roots.

From the results of systematic feeding trials with mixtures of seeds alone and the same with single and multiple purified food additions, and the same type of experiment using certain of the tubers and root foods in place of the seeds, it is shown that all these classes of foodstuffs resemble one another in all respects except in the high content of water in the tubers and roots. In the dry state they are all much like the seeds, but there is one minor difference which should be mentioned. The most important difference lies in the character of the nitrogenous compounds. In the seeds the nitrogen is almost all contained in the form of true protein. In the tubers and edible roots most of it is in the form of much simpler compounds, a part being the same amino-acids which are derived from proteins on digestion.

It is possible to prepare diets derived solely from vegetable products which will nourish an animal during growth and throughout life in a very satisfactory manner, but it is a surprisingly difficult task to prepare for the omnivera, an adequate diet composed entirely of food-stuffs of plant origin. While many of the seeds contain nothing of a detrimental character, many of the leaves, when eaten, undoubtedly do introduce into the body substances which have more or less injurious effects. The nature of these cannot be stated at the present time, but the possibility that there may be an injurious effect brought about by prolonged administration of such bodies as the tannins, the glucosides and oxalic acid, certain organic bases which in some cases resemble certain of the alkaloids, and in some leaves the presence of alkaloids which are highly active pharmacologically, can easily account for the fact that with all rations of strictly vegetable origin one would not have optimum nutrition. McCollum and Simmonds have in a long list of trials with mixtures of leaves and seeds been unable to secure the optimum of well-being in omnivorous animals. *It is worthy of the greatest emphasis that in our hundreds of trials with diets derived entirely from vegetable sources, we have not succeeded in producing optimum results in the nutrition of an omnivorous animal the rat.* Certain of the animals which we have restricted to foods of plant origin, have done so well that we should in the absence of much experience with diets of excellent quality, have considered them to be normal in every respect. It should be emphasized that the average performance of a group of people or animals living upon a *varied diet* cannot safely be assumed to represent the best of which they are capable. In the study of diets the author and his colleagues have kept constantly in mind the best results we have ever seen in the nutrition of animals, as exemplified in rapidity of growth, ultimate size attained, number of young produced, and the success with which these were reared, and have attempted to assign to every experimental group its legitimate place on a scale of performance, which has complete failure to either grow or long remain alive as the one extreme, and the optimum of which the animal is capable as the other.

In connection with the statement which has just been made regarding the strict vegetarian diet, that it does not, so far as has been observed, induce the best results in the nutrition of the omnivora, it should be added that in human dietary practice what is generally designated as vegetarianism is in reality something very different. Many people hold that they are adhering to vegetarian dietary habits, who in reality, take in addition to foods of plant origin, milk or eggs or both. This type of diet will give very much better results than can be secured from the use of vegetable foods alone. Lacto-vegetarianism should not be confuesd with strict vegetarianism. The former is, when the diet is properly planned, the most highly satisfactory plan which can be adopted in the nutrition of man. The latter, if strictly adhered to, is fraught with grave danger unless the diet is planned by one who has extensive and exact knowledge of the special properties of the various food-stuffs employed.

CHAPTER III

It has been pointed out in the preceding chapters that it is not possible to make a diet derived entirely from seeds or seed products, which will adequately nourish an animal during growth, and it may be added that such diets will not even maintain a fully grown animal in a state of health and normal physiological activity over a long period. Without an appropriate supplementing of seed mixtures with the elements, calcium, sodium and chlorine, no appreciable amount of growth has been secured with seed mixtures, in our extensive experience. It was further pointed out that the leaf is a very different thing from the seed, tuber or root, from the dietary standpoint, and these differences in nutritive properties can be correlated with differences in function. The seed is a storage organ of the plant, and is filled with a reserve supply of proteins, carbohydrates, fats and mineral salts. It is in great measure non-living matter, and indeed much of the contents of the seed was never a part of living matter, but only the product of it. In the leaf of the plant we have a tissue which, during life, was very active in the manifestations of the properties of living matter. With these

53

differences in function, it was pointed out, there are found corresponding differences in the dietary values of the two types of foods, the latter being much more nearly complete foods chemically, than are the seeds, tubers and roots.

Let us consider briefly the bearing of these observations on the whole subject of human and animal nutrition. It has been pointed out that for many years the protein and energy value and its digestibility were assumed to determine the value of a food. The chemist is able to determine approximately the amount of protein or rather its content of nitrogen which is taken as a measure of the amount of protein and the fuel value of a food, and by means of experiments on animals, the extent to which a given food is digested and absorbed. He can even tell by a study of the relation between the amounts of oxygen absorbed by the tissues, and the amount of carbon dioxide given off whether the animal is burning sugar or fat in order to obtain its energy. The nitrogen eliminated in the urine serves as a measure of the destruction of protein in the body. Without in the least attempting disparagement of the value of the services of the chemist in the study of the problems of nutrition, it may truthfully be said that both his ordinary and his unusual and most searching methods for the analysis of foodstuffs fail to throw any great amount of light on the value of a food or mixture of foods for inducing growth.

In addition to the cereal grains, wheat, oat, maize, rye, barley and rice, the products of the vegetable garden which supplied leafy vegetables, cabbage, lettuce, spinach, cauliflower, brussels sprouts, chard, celery, various "greens," etc.; roots, such as the radish, turnip and beet; tubers, such as the potato and sweet potato, we have had available as food an abundance of meats and of dairy products. It is not strange that with such a supply of foods it should have been taken for granted that any diet consisting of wholesome foods, combined in such proportions and taken in such quantities as would furnish the amounts of protein and energy which experiments on man and animals had shown to be necessary under specified conditions of living, whether at rest or at work, should prove satisfactory for the maintenance of health in the adult and of normal growth in the young. An appreciation of the fundamental importance of employing proper combinations of foods, was impossible, until the systematic efforts described in the first two chapters, were made to simplify the diet as far as possible, and to derive it from restricted sources. These studies have, when the results were applied to the interpretation of the quality of the diets of man in several parts of the world, revealed the fact that man is frequently failing to make the wisest selection of food. Health and efficiency can be greatly improved by applying the knowledge which we now possess concerning the special properties of several classes of foods, to the selection of the articles which shall make up the daily diet.

The biological method for the analysis of single food-stuffs and mixtures of food-stuffs *has made it evident that the older practice of regarding protein, energy and digestibility as the criteria of the value of a food mixture, must be replaced by a new method of presentation of the subject based upon a biological classification of the food-stuffs, the latter having its foundation in the function of the substance employed in the diet.* Such a method of presentation of the subject of food values offers convincing evidence of the necessity, for the proper selection of food, that dietary reforms are greatly needed in many parts of the world.

There has been much discussion of the relative merits of the vegetarian diet for man as compared with diets largely derived from vegetable foods but more or less liberally supplemented with foods of animal origin. This question has been discussed principally from the point of view of the supposed detrimental effects of a diet containing a high protein content, and the supposed beneficial effects of a sparing consumption of protein, and from the point of view that there are sound ethical reasons why man should abstain from the use of animal foods. The adherents of the latter extreme view have never become numerous, partly because the average individual has not the self-control to enable him to forego the use of meats, milk and eggs, on account of their appetizing qualities, and partly because the chances of one's succeeding in the selection of a strictly vegetarian diet which would maintain such a state of physiological well-being as would make possible the continuation of his line are very small. Concerning the ethical considerations involved in the eating of animal foods, nothing need be said here. The relative merits of the vegetarian as compared with the mixed diet, and the evidence regarding the desirability of taking a low or high protein intake, may next receive our attention.

The most elaborate attempt to test the relative merits of the strictly vegetarian diet as contrasted with the omnivorous type, was made by Slonaker.[1] He fed a group of young rats on a list of 23 vegetable foods, allowing them free choice within limits. For comparison, a similar group were fed the same foods of vegetable origin, but in addition animal food was given in moderate quantities. Since several natural foods, raw or prepared, were offered at a time, and the animals were allowed free choice as to what they should eat, and since no effort was made to keep track of the food consumption, or the relative amounts of the different foods eaten, the results cannot be employed for critical examination except in a limited way. The results are of the greatest interest in showing how far instinct fails to guide an animal in the selection of its food. Slonaker's list of foods included nearly everything which a vegetarian in southern California would be likely to have on his table during the year, and included seeds, the milling products of seeds and leafy vegetables, tubers and roots.

The vegetarian group grew fairly well for a time, but became stunted when they reached a weight of about 60 per cent of the normal adult size. They never increased in size beyond this point. The omnivorous controls grew steadily to what may be regarded as the normal size for the adult. The vegetarians lived, on an average for the entire group, 555 days, whereas the omnivora had an average span of life of 1020 days. The vegetarian rats grew to be approximately half as large, and lived half as long as did their fellows which received animal food. Slonaker drew the conclusion that a strictly vegetarian diet is not suitable for the nourishment of an omnivorous animal, but was unable to say why this should be true.

The results of Slonaker were published in 1912, and just at the time when McCollum and Davis were securing the experimental data which revealed the differences in the growth-promoting power of fats from different sources and which established the fact that a hitherto unsuspected dietary essential existed. They fed their diet of relatively pure foodstuffs described on page 16 with various fats of both animal and vegetable origin and found that no fat which was derived from plant tissues came in the growth-promoting class along with butter fat, the fats of egg yolk, and of the glandular organs. It seemed to McCollum and Davis that the most probable explanation of the results of Slonaker was the absence or shortage in his vegetarian diet of the dietary essential which is furnished so abundantly by butter fat, and which later came to be designated as fat-soluble A and to a low protein intake. With this idea in mind they tried during the summer of 1914 an experiment similar to that of Slonaker's, but modified so as to give the animals a much higher protein content than his rats probably took. It seemed that if Slonaker's vegetarian rats ate liberally of such leaves as cabbage and other leafy vegetables, the protein content of which in the fresh condition does not as a rule exceed 2 per cent, the content of other constituents of the diet in protein might not be high enough to give the entire mixture consumed, a protein content sufficiently high to promote growth at the optimum rate.

McCollum and Davis, therefore, fed their rats a diet which afforded them a choice among the following list of foods: wheat, maize, rye and oat kernels, cooked dry navy beans, peas, wheat germ, corn gluten, wheat gluten, flax-seed oil meal, green clover, green alfalfa leaves, onions and peanuts. It will be observed that in this list there are several vegetable foods having unusually high protein contents. Corn gluten, which is a product of the corn starch manufacture, contains about 25 per cent of protein; wheat gluten, prepared by washing ground wheat free from starch, contains about 86 per cent; flax-seed oil meal, as much as 30 per cent, and wheat germ about 30 per cent of protein. Since animals are known to grow well on many diets containing 15 to 18 per cent of protein, it seemed that with these things to select from, one possible cause of failure in Slonaker's experiments, viz., too low a protein intake, would be avoided. McCollum and Davis had not at that time discovered in the leaf the source of the dietary essential, fat-soluble A, although it is now known that the leafy foods enable the herbivorous animal to thrive on his diet derived entirely from plant tissues. It was then assumed that when both the leaves and so many different seeds as well as the germ was supplied there could be little doubt that everything which a *herbivorous animal* requires was present in the foods supplied.

The rats fed this wide variety of vegetable foods, and with a most liberal supply of protein, duplicated in all respects the results which Slonaker had described. They grew at about half the normal rate for the first few weeks, then became permanently stunted, none ever reaching a size much greater than half that of the average normal adult. The addition of butter fat to the diet of some of these animals failed to benefit them in any noticeable degree. The answer to the question as to why rats do not thrive on such strictly vegetarian food mixtures was not secured from these experiments. It was, however, soon after learned wherein lay the cause of failure of animals so fed.

McCollum, Simmonds and Pitz, began in 1915 a series of feeding experiments in which the diets of rats were derived solely from a mixture of one seed and one dry leaf.[2] In marked contrast to the failure of animals to grow on any mixtures of seeds it was found that in many cases a mixture of a seed with a leaf formed a diet on which considerable growth could be secured. Even polished rice, which as has been already described, requires four types of supplementing, viz, protein, mineral salts, fat-soluble A and water-soluble B, before it becomes dietetically complete, was found to induce fairly good growth when fed with ground alfalfa leaves in the proportion of 60 per cent of the former to 40 per cent of the latter. On this simple monotonous mixture, young rats grew from weaning time to 83 per cent of the normal adult size, and one female even produced two litters of young, both of which were, however, allowed to die within a few days. A mixture of rolled oats, 60 per cent, and alfalfa leaves, 40 per cent, ground together makes a very much better diet. On this simple mixture young rats have been observed to grow to the normal adult size, and to reproduce and rear young. One female reared fourteen out of seventeen young born in three litters. Maize and alfalfa leaf, wheat and alfalfa leaf, are not so satisfactory for the production of growth as is a mixture of rolled oats and alfalfa leaves. Mixtures of the latter leaf with legume seeds, peas and beans, give still poorer results. (Chart 6.) These results made it evident that there is nothing in vegetarianism *per se*, which makes it impossible to nourish an omnivorous animal in a satisfactory manner. It is only necessary to make a proper selection of food-stuffs, and to combine them in the right proportions. In all the experiments described, in which the diet was made up of so simple a mixture as one leaf and one seed, they had not obtained the optimum of growth, reproduction or rearing of young.

It seemed probable that the reason why they did not more closely approximate the optimum in the nutrition of animals restricted to a cereal grain and a leaf, might lie in too low a protein mixture, or a protein mixture which was not of very high biological value. In 1915, McCollum, Simmonds and Pitz [3] fed a group of young rats on a monotonous mixture consisting of maize 50 per cent, alfalfa leaf (dry) 30 per cent, and cooked (dried) peas, subsequently dried, 20 per cent. The three ingredients were ground together so finely that they could not be picked out and eaten separately. This diet induced growth at approximately the normal rate and the production and rearing of a considerable number of young. The young grew up to the full adult size and were successful in the rearing of their offspring. Without ever tasting anything other than this monotonous food mixture, as their sole source of nutriment after the weaning period, this family of rats remained nearly normal, and successfully weaned the young of the fourth generation, with no apparent diminution in vitality. At this point the experiment was discontinued.

The failure of Slonaker's rats to thrive on the vegetarian diet is to be explained on the basis of several faults. In the first place, the diet was of such a nature that the animals could hardly do otherwise than take a rather low protein intake. Secondly, the leaves, which formed the only constituents of the food supply which, contained enough mineral elements to support growth, were fed in the fresh condition. In this form the water content and bulk is so great that it would be practically impossible for an animal whose digestive apparatus is no more capacious than that of an omnivora, to eat a sufficient amount of leaf to correct the inorganic deficiencies of the rest of the mixture, which consisted of grains, seeds, tubers, and root foods. The same physical limitations would likewise determine that the animals would fail to secure enough of the fat-soluble A to supplement the deficiency of all the ingredients of their diet other than the leaves in respect to this factor. This would not form so important a fault as the inorganic deficiencies, but would be an important depressing factor. Thirdly, success or failure would turn in great measure on the extent to which the animals would be guided by instinct in the selection of the proportions of the several types of food-stuffs which was offered them. In the opinion of the author the appetite is by no means so safe a guide for the proper selection of foods as has generally been supposed.

From the results of the experiments just described it was necessary to conclude that the leaf differs from the seed in that it contains in satisfactory amounts the dietary factors which are found in the seeds in too small amounts. These include the three inorganic elements, calcium, sodium and chlorine, the fat-soluble A and a protein supply which supplements at least in some degree the proteins of the seed. These, it will be remembered, are the three and only purified food factors which need be added to each of the seeds singly in order to make it dietetically complete. It is therefore, possible to devise a diet which is derived entirely from vegetable materials which will produce normal growth and the optimum physiological well-being.

At the Iowa Experiment Station, Evvard [4] has conducted extensive experiments of a character which were intended to demonstrate that the appetite and instincts of the hog serve to enable it to make such an adjustment of the relative amounts of the several food-stuffs offered it, as may induce better results in the rate of growth than can be generally secured when the adjustment is made by the feeder, and the mixture of the ingredients of the ration are offered in a form which admitted of no choice by the animal. The data secured in many trials seem to show that there is some basis for the belief that this element of selection by the animal itself is worth taking advantage of. It should be mentioned that, as a rule, in all these trials the animals were given a choice of only three foods, one of these being a cereal grain, another, a protein-rich food and a third a plant leaf. In some experiments a salt mixture was made available. The reasons for the employment of the leaf as a never failing constituent of the food supply of the growing pig could not have been explained before the studies of McCollum and his co-workers, with simplified diets and with diets restricted as to source to a single food-stuff, and until the latter had been fed with single and multiple food additions to ascertain the exact nature of the dietary faults of each. In connection with the types of diets employed by Evvard it should be mentioned that in case the animal ate fairly liberally of all the food-stuffs offered him, a serious mistake would be hardly made, since the proportions of the several constituents eaten could be varied to a considerable degree and growth still take place. In the case of the mixture of maize 50 per cent, alfalfa leaves 30 and peas 20, described above (Chart 7) it has been found that for the rat these are the best proportions in which these three ingredients can be mixed for the promotion of growth and reproduction. It has been further established that using these three food-stuffs, a moderate amount of growth may be secured, but few, if any, young will ever be produced if the mixture fed contains more than 50 per cent or less than 20 per cent of alfalfa leaf. The importance of combining the natural foods in the right proportions is easily seen from these results.   It is interesting to note further, that shifting the proportions of maize, peas and leaf in this mixture over a range of 20 per cent does not materially ·change the protein content, or indeed, the chemical composition of the food mixture in any way, to a degree that could be expected to make so great a difference in the state of nutrition of the animals as is actually observed.

There are now available the results of a very extensive series of feeding trials in which the rations were made up of one seed, one leaf and one legume (pea, bean) in various proportions.   These have failed to reveal any mixture which is quite the equal of the first ration of this type ever employed, viz., that composed of maize 50, alfalfa leaf 30 and peas 20 per cent.   It is, of course, easily possible that better mixtures of vegetable foods may be found by further search, but these results show very definitely that for the omnivorous type of animal, whose digestive tract is so constituted that the consumption of large volumes of leafy foods is not possible, it is by no means a simple matter, if indeed possible, to derive the diet entirely from the vegetable foods, and secure the optimum of well-being.   The data afforded by the experiments described form a demonstration of the fact that wide variety is of little value as a safeguard to nutrition.   Chemical analysis, no matter how thorough, fails to throw much light upon the dietary value of a food-stuff.   The only way in which the problems of nutrition can be solved is through numerous properly planned feeding experiments, but such studies were not possible before the solution of the problem of successfully feeding mixtures of purified food-stuffs. These studies led to the formulation of an adequate working hypothesis regarding what factors operate to make an adequate diet, and made possible the interpretation of the cause of success or of failure with diets of the complexity employed in daily life. It will be shown later that the consumption of milk and its products forms the greatest factor for the protection of mankind, in correcting the faults in his otherwise vegetarian and meat diet.

The fact, that although the cereal grains each contain every inorganic element which is contained in an animal body, and every one which is a necessary constituent of the diet, but in too small amounts in the case of three of them, to enable the animals to grow, revealed the mineral constituents of the diet in a new and important light. The animal is sensitive to either the actual amounts of certain of the mineral elements in the food mixture, or to the relationships among them. Sidney Ringer was led in 1891 to his description of Ringer's solution, as the result of the observations in physiology, that muscle behaves more nearly normally in solutions containing certain salts in definite proportions. Ringer's solution contains, for each 100 molecules of sodium chloride, two molecules of calcium chloride and two to one molecules of potassium chloride, together with a trace of a magnesium salt.   Loeb,[5] Howell [6] and others had described many experiments showing the profound effects upon the subsequent development of the eggs of varying in certain ways the composition of the salt solutions in which unfertilized eggs of certain marine animals were kept.   In this way the earliest stages of development which are ordinarily observed only in the fertilized egg, could be caused to take place in eggs into which no sperm had entered.   In the nutrition of the higher animals, it had never been made clear how dependent the organism is on the rate at which the blood stream receives mineral nutrient.   The fact that the cereal grains are too low in three inorganic elements to admit of growth, made it clear that food packages just as they come from the hand of Nature, are not necessarily so constituted as to promote health.

CHAPTER IV

THE FOODS OF ANIMAL ORIGIN

It is well known from common observation that milk, when it serves as the sole food of the infant, serves to keep it growing normally and in good health over a long period. There has occasionally arisen a discussion as to whether milk is a suitable food for the adult, and as to whether it is the "ideal" food. Milk, like the cereal grains and most other natural foods, contains all the essential food elements, and human experience teaches us that the proportions in which they occur in this product are much more satisfactory than in many other natural foods. Animals grow well on milk, but it is not easy to find even complex food mixtures of vegetable foods which will support optimum nutrition in the omnivora during growth.

Milk is deficient in iron, as is shown by chemical analysis. It has long been known that there is deposited in the spleen of the new-born animal a reserve supply of iron, which ordinarily suffices to tide it over the suckling period. Ordinary drinking water almost always contains small amounts of iron, and this doubtless aids in some degree in preventing iron starvation in the infant.

That milk is a complete food, capable of supplying all the nutrients necessary for the prolonged maintenance of growth, health and the ability to produce and rear young, was shown by an experiment conducted by the author at the Wisconsin Experiment Station. A female pig was removed from its mother, which was still nursing it at the weight of 17 pounds. She had doubtless eaten of the mother's ration to some extent but her principle food had been her mother's milk. After removal from the mother, this pig was confined in a pen having a board floor, and was fed nothing but milk during a period of 17 months. During the first few months only whole milk was fed, but later it was necessary to replace this in part by skim milk. The animal weighed 406 pounds at the age of thirteen months. At this age she produced eight living and two dead pigs, and successfully brought the young to an average weight of seventeen pounds. She had access to wood shavings, and ate some of them. There can be no doubt that the milk which she consumed was enriched to some *extent with iron* by being in contact with cans having part of the surface free from tin. City drinking water was also furnished and this contained appreciable amounts of iron. The animal must have been able to conserve its limited iron supply in a very efficient manner.

Milk is, therefore, capable of nourishing the pig during many months, with no other modification or additions than small amounts of iron. That it is best to select milk as a monotonous and restricted diet during adult life, no one familiar with the principles of nutrition would maintain. Milk is, however, without doubt our most important food-stuff. *This is true, because the composition of milk is such that when used in combination with other food-stuffs of either animal or vegetable origin, it corrects their dietary deficiencies.* Combinations of equal weights of milk and one of the cereal grains give excellent results in the nutrition of animals during growth, and grain mixtures supplemented with milk support well in adult life the function of reproduction and rearing of young. This is because of the excellent quality of its proteins, the peculiar composition of its inorganic content and the remarkable content of the dietary essential, fat-soluble A, in the fats of milk. Milk, like nearly all of the other natural foods, contains a great abundance of the second dietary essential of unknown chemical nature, water-soluble B.

The extraordinary value of the proteins of milk has been abundantly demonstrated by experiment. McCollum [1] conducted a series of experiments with growing pigs to determine the extent to which they could retain the protein of the food for the construction of new body protein. The pig was selected because it is necessary in such studies to work with an animal whose growth impulse is as great as possible. Only with such species is it to be expected that the animal will utilize the proteins for growth to the maximum extent made possible by the chemical character of the food protein. The human infant has but little growth impulse because its period of infancy is long and the adult size not great as compared with the size at birth. A comparison of the human infant with the rat and the young pig (swine) in their capacity to grow in early life is of interest. The human infant weighs not far from seven pounds at birth, and during the first year of life is ordinarily able to multiply its initial body weight by three, for the average weight at one year is about twenty-one pounds. We may feed it human milk the entire time, or unmodified cows' milk during the greater part of the year, without in any important degree modifying its rate of growth. In the latter case, we should be supplying it with perhaps double the amount of protein that it would receive were it fed human milk, since the latter contains on an average about 1.6 per cent and the former about 3.5 per cent of protein.

In marked contrast to the feeble capacity of the human infant to store new tissue and increase in size, stand the rat and the pig. The rat at birth weighs about 4.83 grams, and contains about 0.064 grams of nitrogen. At 280 days of age the male should weigh about 280 grams, and if moderately fat will contain about 8.5 grams of nitrogen. The rat is able, therefore, in a period of 280 days to multiply its initial body weight by about 55, and its initial body nitrogen content (protein) by 133.

The newborn pig weighing two pounds will contain about 134 grams of dry matter and 11.9 grams of nitrogen. In 280 days it may, if properly fed, reach a weight of 300 pounds. It would then have a nitrogen content of not less than 2407 grams. These changes in size entail a multiplication of the initial body weight by 150 and of the initial body nitrogen content by 202. The farm pig is apparently the most rapidly growing species of land animals.

Such considerations determined the selection of the pig as a subject for the test of the biological value of the proteins of the various natural food-stuffs. The plan involved keeping the animal for a period of several days on a diet free from protein, but containing sufficient starch to cover the energy requirements. When the nitrogen elimination in the urine reached a constant low level which represented the irreducible minimum, resulting from the "wear and tear" of the tissues, the animal was fed a diet containing protein derived solely from a single grain, or other single food-stuff. A record was kept of the intake of the element nitrogen, and of the daily loss of this element through the excreta, and from these records the percentage retained for growth was obtained. Similar experiments were carried out using milk as the sole source of protein. The following table summarizes the results obtained.

Source of protein	Per cent of ingested protein retained
Corn	20.0
Wheat	23.0
Oats (rolled)	26.0
Milk	63.0

The figures in the table are averages of a considerable number of results and represent the general trend of the data. The experimental periods varied from 30 to 60 days. There can be no doubt that the proteins of milk are far superior to those of any foods derived from vegetable sources.

The problem of determining the relative values of the proteins of the different foods *when fed singly*, supplemented with purified food additions that their dietary deficiencies were made good, was approached in a different way by McCollum and Simmonds.[2] Rats were fed diets in which the protein was all furnished by a single natural food-stuff, but the plane of protein intake was varied from very low to higher intakes, in order to determine what was the lowest per cent of protein in the food mixture which would just suffice to maintain an animal without loss of body weight. The rations consisted of the following substances:

Seed	Amount to give the protein intake desired
Growth-promoting fat (butter-fat)	5.0 per cent
Suitably constituted salt mixtures	3 to 5 per cent
Agar-agar (to furnish indigestible matter)	2.0 per cent
Dextrin	To make 100 per cent.

The results showed that there are indeed very great differences in the amounts of protein from different seeds, which are necessary to maintain an animal without loss of body weight. The results for the more important seeds used as human foods are summarized in the following table.

TABLE SHOWING THE LOWEST PLANE OF PROTEIN INTAKE DE-
RIVED FROM A SINGLE SEED WHICH JUST SUFFICES TO MAIN-
TAIN AN ANIMAL IN BODY WEIGHT, WHEN THE FACTORS
OTHER THAN PROTEIN ARE PROPERLY CONSTITUTED

Source of Protein   Plane of Protein Necessary for Maintenance

Source of Protein	Plane of Protein Necessary for Maintenance
Milk	3.0 per cent of food mixture [3]
Oat (rolled)	4.5 " " " " "
Millet seed	4.5 " " " " "
Maize	6.0 " " " " "
Wheat	6.0 " " " " "
Polished rice	6.0 " " " " "
Flax seed	8.0 " " " " "
Navy bean	12.0 " " " " "
Pea	12.0 " " " " "

These maintenance experiments were of three to six months' duration.

The data obtained with the pig is seen to be in harmony in a general way with those obtained with the rat, and help to substantiate the view which is supported by all the evidence available, viz: that from the chemical standpoint, the dietary requirements of one species of animal are the same as those of another. That there are great differences in the physical characters of the diet which suffice for, or are required by certain species as contrasted with others, is a matter of common observation. The ruminants actually require coarse herbage as a part of their food, in order that the alimentary tract may function properly, whereas such physical properties in the diet of the omnivora are wholly out of place beyond very limited amounts.

In considering the value of milk as a constituent of the diet it should be borne in mind that with respect to the protein factor it may enhance the value of the proteins of the remainder of the food. It may supply in relative abundance those amino-acids which are present in such small amounts that they form the first, second, etc., limiting factors in determining the value of the protein for growth or maintenance, as well as by the direct addition to the food mixture, of the intrinsically good proteins of the milk.

When taken as the sole food supply by the adult, milk is very liable to produce constipation and because of its high protein content, may lead to the excessive development of putrefactive bacteria in the intestine. The cages of rats fed solely on milk develop an offensive odor. The addition of carbohydrate, such as starch or certain of the sugars, tend to cause the disappearance of the obnoxious flora from the alimentary tract, and the development, instead, of types which do not produce injurious decomposition products in their action on proteins.

Meats.—The muscle tissue of an animal consists of highly specialized tissue whose chief function is to produce mechanical work through contraction. It is in addition a storage organ in which glycogen, a form of starch, and also fats are stored as reserve foods. It contains but little of cellular structures in the sense that the glandular organs, such as the liver, kidney, pancreas, etc, do. Chemical analysis shows the muscle to consist, aside from the reserve food-stuffs, principally of water, protein and salts. The glandular organs yield a high content of nucleic acid, while the muscle tissue yields but little in pro-portion to its weight. The inorganic content of the muscle tissue resembles that of the seed of the plant, rather than the leaf both in amount and in the rel-ative proportions among the elements.

Corresponding with the specialized function, and the peculiarities in composition just mentioned, we find that its dietary properties are comparable with the seed rather than the leaf. In fact; muscle tissue differs markedly from the seed in only one respect, when considered as a food-stuff, viz., in the quality of its proteins. These are distinctly better than those of the seeds with which investigations have been conducted. The inorganic content must be supplemented by the same inorganic additions as the seed, and the muscle proves to be relatively poor in its content of the unidentified dietary essential fat-soluble A, as compared with such foods as milk, egg yolk and the leaves of plants.

Since the inorganic part of muscle resembles that of the seed, except that the latter is poorer in iron and it is low in its content of fat-soluble A, it does not supplement the seeds in an appreciable degree other than with respect to the protein factor. It follows, therefore, that we should not expect to secure growth and normal nutrition with mixtures of seeds, and meat and experimental trials demonstrate that this is the case.---Mixtures of meat (muscle) and seeds require to be supplemented with respect to sodium. calcium and chlorine, just as do seed mixtures alone[4]. The fat-soluble A content of such mixtures, unless millet seed is one of the seeds present to the extent of 25 per cent, must be increased by suitable additions before the optimum nutrition can be attained, and the animals can successfully bear the strain of reproduction and lactation. Meats are, therefore, but partial supplementary foods when employed with the seeds or the products prepared from seeds, such as wheat flour, corn meal, polished rice, etc. Such diets can be partially corrected by the liberal use of leafy vegetables, but better by the use of the latter along with milk.

The pronounced deficiencies of muscle tissue as a food-stuff, naturally suggests the question of the reason for the success of the nutrition of the strictly carnivorous animals. The explanation is found in the order in which such creatures select the parts of the carcasses of their prey. The larger carnivoræ, after striking down an animal, immediately open the large veins of the neck and suck blood as long as it flows. Their second choice of tissues is the liver, and

following this the other glandular organs.   Muscle
tissue is only eaten after these have been consumed.
With such a selection the animal secures eveıything
which it needs for its nutrition except a sufficient
amount of calcium, and this is obtained through
gnawing off the softer parts of the extremities of the
bones.   The failure of many carnivora to thrive when
confined in zoos, it probably the result of their being
fed too largely upon muscle tissue and bones.   They
should be supplied with an abundance of the glandular organs and with blood to make their diet complete.   With rats McCollum, Simmonds and Parsons
have observed fairly satisfactory growth on equal
parts of muscle tissue (round steak) and dried
blood,   whereas either of these alone cannot induce
growth.[4]

The Glandular Organs.—The liver and kidney
may serve as typical examples of the glandular organs which are employed as foods.   There are certain organs of internal secretion, such as the thy-
roid, and suprarenal glands which elaborate products
which are highly active pharmacological agents, and
the liberal use of these glands as food would lead to
disastrous consequences.   The glands contain but little of the inorganic elements in which the seeds are
deficient.   Their proteins are probably of excellent
quality, but have not yet been carefully investigated.
The glands consist[1] largely of actively functioning
cells, having specialized functions, and accordingly
they prove to contain a more liberal amount of both

the fat-soluble A and water-soluble B than does the muscle. In respect to the former of the unidentified dietary essentials the glandular organs surpass the seeds in value.[4] From this description it will be seen that the glandular organs approximate more closely complete foods than does the muscle, but it is likewise apparent that these tissues do not form efficient supplements for the seeds and their products.

Eggs.—The egg contains all the chemical complexes necessary for the formation of the chick during incubation. The egg is therefore to be expected to furnish everything which is needed for the nutrition of a mammal, for as has been already stated, the evidence all supports the belief that the chemical requirements of one species are the same as another. The egg is indeed a complete food, but not one which produces the optimum results when employed as the sole source of nutriment. Aside from the calcium content of the white and yolk of the egg, which is much lower than that of milk, the contents of the egg resemble milk in a general way in nutritional value. The high content of milk sugar in the latter, and the almost complete absence of carbohydrate from the egg, cause them to differ considerably in the physiological results which they produce on animals when each is fed as the sole source of nutriment. Egg, when fed alone, encourages much more than milk the development of putrefactive organisms in the alimentary tract. The shell of the egg consists principally of calcium carbonate, and during incubation this is to some extent dissolved and absorbed for the formation of the chick. When eggs serve as human food the shells are discarded. There are distinct differences in the chemical natures of the constituents of eggs as contrasted with milk. The principal protein of egg yolk, like that of milk, contains phosphorus, but the fats of milk are phosphorus free, whereas phosphorized fats (*e. g.,* lecithins) are very abundant in egg fats. There is an abundance of lactose in milk, whereas the egg contains but a trace of sugar. These differences have little, if any, dietary significance. The yolk is especially rich in both the fat-soluble A and water-soluble B. *With the exception of milk the foods of animal origin do not supplement completely the dietary deficiencies of the seeds and their products.*

† We are now able to make certain generalizations of fundamental importance regarding the types of combinations of the natural food-stuffs which may be expected to give good results in the nutrition of an animal.

(1) Seed mixtures, no matter how complex, or from what seeds they are derived, will never induce optimum nutrition.

Seeds with tubers, or seeds with tubers, roots and meat (muscle) will in all cases fail to even approximate the optimum in the nutrition of an animal during growth.

(2) The only successful combinations of natural

foods or milled products for the nutrition of an animal are:

    (a) Combinations of seeds, or other milled products, tubers and roots, either singly or collectively taken with sufficient amounts of the leaves of plants.

    (b) Combinations of the food-stuffs enumerated under (a) taken along with a sufficient amount of milk to make good their deficiencies.

Milk and the leaves of plant are to be regarded as protective foods and should never be omitted from the diet. Milk is a better protective food than are the leaves, when used in appropriate amounts.

It should be appreciated that not all diets which conform to the requirements laid down in the above generalizations, will give equally good results. This is especially true of diets of the type under (2). Chart 6 shows the great differences in the food values of a few mixtures of seeds and leaves. It can be stated definitely, however, that diets which are not made up according to the second plan, will never be satisfactory.

CHAPTER V

It has been pointed out that in the year 1911 Funk took up the study of the disease beri-beri. He made use of the observation of Eijkman, that the symptoms could be produced experimentally in birds by feeding them exclusively upon polished rice for two to four weeks, whereas birds remain for much longer periods in a state of health when fed exclusively upon the unpolished grain. He also made use of the observation of Fraser and Stanton, that an alcoholic extract of rice polishings would effect a "cure" of polyneuritic birds. Funk made numerous elaborate and painstaking attempts to separate the "curative" substance, and wrote extensively on what he believed to be "deficiency" diseases. Under this term he included beri-beri, scurvy, pellagra and rickets. Hopkins discovered that small additions of milk to food mixtures composed of purified protein, carbohydrate, fats and inorganic salts, rendered them capable of inducing growth, whereas without such additions no growth could be secured. The effects were out of all proportion to the energy, or protein value of the added milk, and he suggested the existence of "accessory" food-stuffs, which are required in but small amounts, and which are absent from the mixtures of purified food-stuffs, which fail to promote growth. To the supposed "curative" substances, the presence of which in the diet prevents the development of several syndromes enumerated, Funk gave the collective name "vitamines." Thus he distinguished an antineuritic "vitamine," an antiscorbutic "vitamine," etc. These supposed substances have since been variously designated as "growth substances," "growth determinants," "food hormones," "accessory" food substances, etc.

McCollum and Davis through their studies with diets of purified food-stuffs, pointed out that it was highly probable that there are essential in the diet but two substances rather than groups of substances of unknown chemical nature, and it was shown, as has been pointed out, that one of them is associated with certain fats, while the other is never found with the isolated fats of either animal or vegetable origin. McCollum and Kennedy [1] suggested that they be provisionally called fat-soluble A and water-soluble B, because of their characteristic solubility in fats and in water respectively.

The above terms, except the last two, are misnomers. The word accessory, carries the idea that the substances in question are dispensable. Condiments may be desirable, but they can be dispensed with and are properly designated as accessory food substances. An indispensable food complex cannot properly be designated by this term. "Vitamine" is objectionable, because the prefix *vita* connotes an importance of these dietary essentials greater than other equally indispensable constituents of the diet, such as certain of the amino-acids which play a rôle in protein metabolism. The ending *amine* has a definite and specific meaning in organic chemistry, being used to designate a compound derived from ammonia by the substitution of one or more of its hydrogen atoms by various organic radicals. Any substance to be properly designated as amine must contain the element nitrogen. There is no evidence that either of these unidentified dietary essentials is an amine, and indeed fat-soluble A probably contains no nitrogen, for it is especially abundant in butter fat, and the latter is practically free from this element.

"Food hormones" is an objectionable term, because all the evidence available indicates that both the fat-soluble A and water-soluble B are never-failing constituents of the cells of both animal and plant tissues. They have nothing in common with the hormones. The latter are chemical substances which are formed in the body by special tissues and contributed to the blood stream where they cause the stimulation of certain other tissues to physiological activity. They are chemical messengers, while the substances under discussion are food complexes, apparently necessary for all the living cells of the body. It has been pointed out that the content of both of these two dietary essentials appears to run parallel to the content of cellular elements in the food-stuffs, regardless of their source.

"Growth substances" and "growth determinants" are not good terms for the reason that the substances in question are just as essential for the maintenance of a full grown animal in a state of health as they are for the support of growth in the young. Furthermore, in actual experience, rations are found in which the content of one or more essential amino-acids are present in such amounts that they form the limiting factor which *determines* the value of the ration. It is easy to prepare a food mixture in which any one of the eight or nine essential inorganic elements which the diet must furnish, will be so low as to prevent the growth of an animal even though the food is otherwise of satisfactory character. In one case the addition of a suitable sodium compound or in another a calcium or a potassium salt might induce growth, and these elements might, with just as much propriety, be called "growth determinants" as to apply this term to one of the still unidentified food essentials. The term might fittingly be applied to any of the indispensable components of the diet, such as certain of the amino-acids, which result from the digestion of the proteins.

All natural food-stuffs, such as the seeds of plants, the leafy vegetables, fruits, roots, tubers, meats, eggs and milk, contain certain amounts of all the substances which are indispensable components of

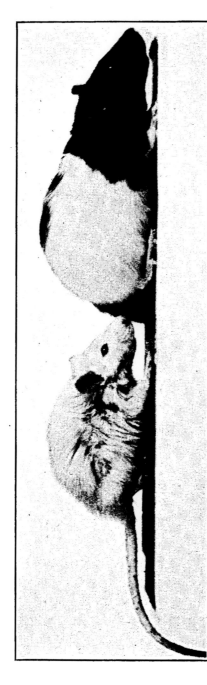

FIG. 5.—The rations of these two rats from weaning time were exactly alike except in the character of the fat which they contained. The one on the left was given 5 per cent of sun-flower seed oil. The one on the right was given 1.5 per cent of butter fat. Butter fat, egg yolk fats and the leaves of plants, contain a dietary essential, the chemical nature of which is still unknown, which is necessary for growth or the maintenance of health. This substance is known as fat-soluble A, and is not found in any fats or oils of vegetable origin. A lack of this substance in the diet causes the development of a peculiar eye disease known as xerophthalmia.

the diet. There is, however, great variation in the *quality* of the different foods with respect to the several factors. Some contain much protein, others little, and a similar variation with respect to other constituents is found. The special properties of the several groups of food-stuffs have been described in Chapters III and IV.

The best sources of fat-soluble A are whole milk, butter fat and egg yolk fats and the leaves of plants. The seeds of plants contain less and those products derived from the endosperm of the seed are very poor in this substance. Such food-stuffs as bolted flour, degerminated corn meal, polished rice, starch, glucose and the sugars from milk, cane, and beet are practically free from the fat-soluble A. The specific result of a lack of a sufficient amount of this substance in the diet is the development of a condition of the eyes which appears to be rightly classed as a type of xerophthalmia. The eyes become swollen so badly that they are opened with difficulty or not at all. The cornea becomes inflamed, and unless the missing dietary essential is supplied, blindness speedily results. Osborne and Mendel [2] have also noted this condition in experimental animals and its relief by feeding butter fat. The introduction into the diet of 5 or more per cent of butter fat will cause prompt recovery in cases where the animals are within a few days of death. Complete recovery takes place within two weeks if the sight has not been destroyed. The normal condition of the eyelids can be restored even after the sight is gone and the cornea has faded.

When the diet consists principally of one of the cereal grains such as the wheat, oat or corn kernel, or even a mixture of these, and it is satisfactorily supplemented with respect to the inorganic elements in which they are deficient, viz., calcium, sodium and chlorine, and their proteins are enhanced in value by the addition of a protein of good quality, animals restricted to such a food supply may long escape the onset of this disease. The seeds are not entirely lacking in the substance, fat-soluble A. They contain, especially the wheat and corn kernels, about half the amount required to maintain an animal in a state of health. If the seeds or their mixtures are supplemented with respect to but a single dietary factor, e. g. inorganic salts, but the protein content is left of relatively low biological value, the debilitating effects of the low value of the food mixture in the two dietary factors (protein and fat-soluble A) simultaneously will hasten the onset of xerophthalmia.[3] When judging the effects of the diet on an animal, it is necessary to take into account the fact that the diet is a complex thing, and that if it is properly constituted with respect to all factors but one an animal may tolerate it without apparent injury whether the fault lies in one or another of the essential components. The value of one component may fall well below that which will lead to serious malnutrition, when a second dietary factor is likewise poor.

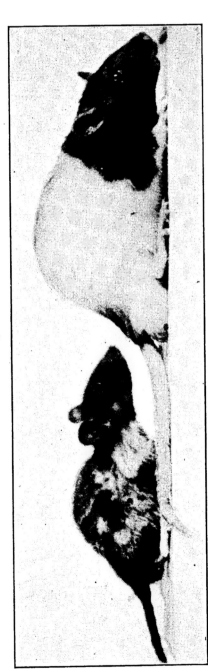

FIG. 6.—From weaning time the rations of these two rats were identical except in the character of the fats which they contained. The rat on the right was given 1.5 per cent of butter fat in its diet, while the one on the left received 5 per cent of bleached cottonseed oil. The former grew at the normal rate, while the latter remained stunted, and suffered loss of hair and emaciation. The small rats in Figures 5 and 6 had not yet developed xerophthalmia when photographed.

The idea should not be entertained that butter fat is the only food which supplies the fat-soluble A. If the diet contains a liberal amount of milk, eggs, glandular organs or the leaves of plants, it will, if otherwise satisfactorily constituted, prevent the onset of the eye disease. The seeds and seed products, such as wheat flour (bolted), degerminated corn meal, polished rice, starch, the sugars, syrups, tubers, roots, such as the radish, beet, carrot, turnip, etc., and also the muscle tissue of animals, such as ham, steak, chops, etc., do not contain enough of the fat-soluble A to be classed as important sources of this dietary essential. The tubers and roots appear to be somewhat richer in it than are the seeds.[4] In the form in which they are ordinarily eaten, as mashed or baked potato, baked sweet potato, fresh or creamed radish, cooked carrots, beets or creamed turnips, the water content of the dish as served is so high that the amount of solids eaten is not a very high per cent of the total food supply, and the protective action is correspondingly limited. In America, however, potatoes are seldom eaten without the addition of butter. The vegetable fats and oils such as olive oil, cottonseed oil, peanut and cocoanut oils, although good energy yielding foods, do not furnish this dietary essential. The body fats of animals such as lard, beef fat, etc., are not important sources of the fat-soluble A.

McCollum and his co-workers have repeatedly observed in experimental animals the type of xerophthalmia of dietary origin which has been described above.   They have many times rescued animals from the threshold of death by the addition of butter fat to the diets of the animals which were suffering from the disease which was brought about by a lack of a sufficient amount of the fat-soluble A in their food.   It is important to inquire whether or not this disease has ever occurred in man.   It is not easy to decide from the descriptions, in the clinical literature, of the eye troubles of poorly nourished peoples in various parts of the world, which are of the peculiar type with which we are now dealing, and which are due to other causes.   Soreness of the eyes is common among many primitive peoples. Herdlika [5] describes severe eye troubles among the American Indians of the southwest, and attributed them to too great exposure to strong sunlight.   Infection of the eyes is common among many peoples, and the clinician, not being aware of the existence of a pathological condition of the eyes due to faulty diet, would, of course, be inclined to attribute such conditions to other causes.

There are several instances of the occurrence of conditions described in the literature as xerophthalmia, which seem to be beyond question, cases in which the disease has occurred in man as the result of specific starvation for the dietary essential, fat-soluble A.   Mori [6] in Japan described in 1904, fourteen hundred cases of xerophthalmia among children in a time of food shortage.   He describes the condi-

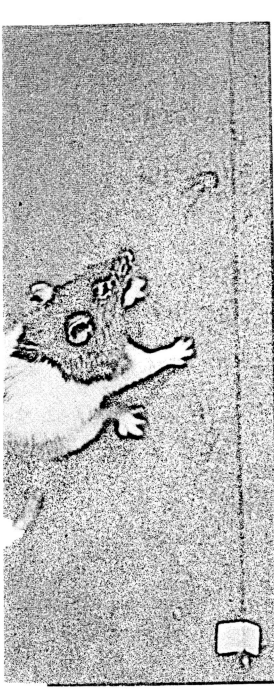

FIG. 7.—This photograph illustrates the condition of the eyes of animals suffering from xerophthalmia of dietary origin, brought on by a lack of the dietary essential, fat-soluble A, in the food supply. In its early stages there is prompt recovery when 5 or more per cent of butter fat or a suitable amount of other food rich in this dietary essential is added to the food. Unless relieved by the administration of the missing food complex, blindness always results, and the animal dies. Compare these eyes with those of normal rats at the right in Figures 5 and 6.

tion in a manner which agrees closely with that which McCollum and Simmonds have observed in animals whose diets were lacking in a sufficient amount of fat-soluble A. The evidence that he was dealing with this disease is made almost conclusive by the fact that he states that feeding chicken livers effected a cure. It has been already mentioned that the glandular organs contain the fat-soluble A in fairly liberal amounts. The Japanese have, as a rule, no dairy products. Their diet consists of seeds and seed products, roots, tubers, leaves and meats, principally fish. Their principal sources of the dietary factor in question are the leafy vegetable and eggs, the former of which in normal times they consume much larger amounts than do the peoples of most parts of Europe and America. Shortage of food will occur usually owing to drought, and the first products which fail are the green vegetables, and accordingly the dietary essential which would be least abundant would be the fat-soluble A. Mori attributed the xerophthalmia to fat starvation. It seems highly probable, however, that a lack of fat was not in itself the cause of the disease, but rather the lack of the unidentified dietary essential which is associated with certain fats, but is not furnished by any of the isolated fats of vegetable origin, although it is present in plant tissues where these contain cellular structures. Mori states that the disease does not occur among fisher folk.

Bloch [7] has recently described forty cases of severe

necrosis of the cornea with ulceration, in the vicinity of Copenhagen. The children had been fed nearly fat-free separator skim milk, and were atrophic or dystrophic and anemic. He attributed the disorder to fat starvation, since the children responded with recovery when fed breast milk, or in the case of older ones, with whole milk mixtures and to codliver oil administration. The recovery, it will be noted, followed the feeding of those substances which are good sources of the fat-soluble A.

Czerny and Keller [8] describe a similar condition of the eyes in children suffering from malnutrition as the result of being restricted to a cereal diet.

It seems certain that these cases of xerophthalmia should be looked upon as a "deficiency disease" not hitherto recognized in its proper relation to diet. It is not a fat starvation, but, if it be the same condition which McCollum and Simmonds have definitely shown to be readily relieved in its early stages by the administration of such foods as contain liberal amounts of fat-soluble A, it would not be relieved by feeding with vegetable fats in any amounts. Milk, eggs, leafy vegetables and the glandular organs, are the foods which serve to protect against a shortage of this indispensable dietary component. This type of xerophthalmia is analogous to beri-beri, in that it is due to the lack of a specific substance in the diet. Beri-beri and xerophthalmia are according to McCollum and Simmonds, the only diseases referable to faulty diet, which are to be explained in this way.

Beri-beri is a disease common in the Orient among peoples who limit their diet largely to polished rice and fish. It has, in recent years, been described in Laborador owing to excessive consumption of bolted flour,[9] and in Brazil among laborers whose diets were of varied character, but not judiciously chosen.[10] Its most striking characteristic is a general paralysis, and it is frequently referred to, especially when produced experimentally in animals, as polyneuritis.

The disease was first produced in animals by Eijkman [11] in 1897. He discovered that when pigeons and chickens were restricted to a diet of polished rice, they steadily lost weight and in time came to manifest all the essential symptoms characteristic of beri-beri in man. In pigeons the disease usually appears in two or three weeks. He found that feeding rice polishings would produce a relief of the symptoms. This result suggested that there was lacking from polished rice, something which was necessary for the maintenance of health in the bird, and that that something was present in the rice polishings. This was the first experimental evidence that there is necessary in the diet substances other than proteins, carbohydrates, fats and inorganic salts.

The observations of Eijkman attracted but little attention until Funk [12] took up the study of beri-beri in 1910. Fraser and Stanton had, as early as 1907, employed alcoholic extracts of rice polishings for the cure of experimental polyneuritis. Funk made numerous studies directed toward the isolation and study of the substance which exerts the curative effect, and developed in his writings the well-known "vitamine" hypothesis. This hypothesis postulated the existence of a similar protective substance for each of the diseases scurvy, pellagra and rickets, in addition to that which in the normal diets protects against beri-beri.

Funk had experimental evidence in support of his theory only in the case of beri-beri. The evidence that the other diseases which he included in the category of "deficiency" diseases are due to the lack of specific.complexes, was of the nature of clinical observations, rather than well controlled experiments. The peculiar value of butter fat was unknown to him, and he classed it among the food substances which contain no "vitamine" because its administration to polyneuritic pigeons produced no beneficial effects.[13] Funk deserves great credit for the evidence which he secured that the amount of the substance which can be extracted from rice polishings, which is necessary to cause the relief of polyneuritis in a pigeon, is exceedingly small. A few milligrams of material which is still contaminated with impurities suffices to bring about relief in a bird which is in a helpless condition and within a few hours of death, and to make it appear like a normal pigeon. The effects seem to be out of all proportion to the amount of substance administered. Funk's studies were confirmed and extended by the important work of Williams.[14]

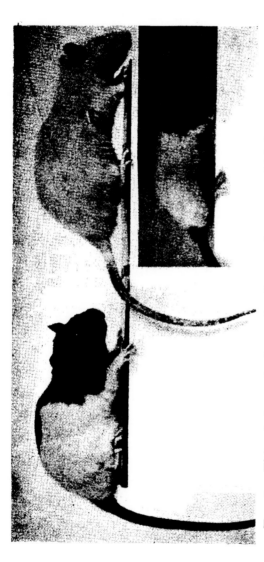

FIG. 8.—This photograph shows the degree of success which has been attained in securing growth, reproduction and rearing of young in an omniverous animal, the rat, with a diet of strictly vegetable origin. The diet is described on page **62**. The data available seems to demonstrate that successful diets of plant origin can be secured only when the leaf of the plant is a prominent constituent of the diet. Those parts of the plant whose functions are those of storage organs (seeds, tubers and roots), do not serve as adequate diets, even when there is a wide variety in the food supply. The leafy structures are so constituted as to correct the deficiencies of mixtures of seeds, tubers and roots.

The albino and her daughter are shown above, and her granddaughter below. Young in the fourth generation were successfully reared, with no apparent diminution in vitality.

There can be no doubt that there are two "deficiency" diseases in the sense in which Funk and his school employed this term. One of these is beri-beri and the other the type of xerophthalmia which McCollum and Simmonds have pointed out as occurring occasionally in man as the result of faulty diet, and have demonstrated to be the same condition which results in animals as the result of specific starvation for the unidentified dietary essential fat-soluble A. It is of the greatest importance to determine whether scurvy, pellagra and possibly rickets are likewise to be attributed to the lack of similar substances of a specific nature in the diet. It has already been mentioned in Chapter II that from a knowledge of the dietary properties of the oat kernel, McCollum and Pitz concluded from a study of experimental scurvy in the guinea pig, that this disease, while referable to faulty diet, does not result from the absence of any special substance from the diet. The evidence upon which this conclusion rests has been touched upon (page 36) and will be next briefly considered.

The oat kernel, when submitted to the biological method of analysis described in the first chapter, was found to contain all the chemical elements and complexes necessary for the promotion of growth and health in a mammal, but not in suitable proportions. Like other seeds it requires certain inorganic additions, and its content of the unidentified fat-soluble A is entirely too small to permit of growth, or to

protect an animal against the eye disease, xerophthalmia.   In addition, its proteins are not comparable in value with those of such foods as milk,
eggs and meats.   The important fact was demonstrated by McCollum, Simmonds and Pitz, that
*if the extracts of natural foods which we have long em-
ployed in our experimental work and which we designate water-soluble B, contain any physiologically indispensable substance other than that which prevents
beri-beri, the oat kernel contains all of these.*   This
follows from the fact that they were able to induce
normal growth and prolonged well-being in animals
fed the oat kernel supplemented *only with purified
food substances,*—viz: protein and inorganic salts,
and a growth-promoting fat.   The latter term
is used to designate a fat containing the fat-
soluble A.

McCollum and Pitz observed that the guinea pig
suffers from scurvy, not only when restricted to a
diet of oats, as stated by Holst, but likewise when fed
oats and all the fresh milk it will consume.   Jackson
and Moore [15] made this observation independently
and described it several months previous, in their
excellent studies of the bacteriology of the digestive
tract and tissues of the guinea pig, after the animals
have developed the disease as the result of an ex-
clusive oat and milk diet.   Milk alone is a complete
food, and suffices for the maintenance of growth and
a good state of nutrition in several species of animals,
such as the rat and swine.   It cannot, therefore, be

lacking in any unidentified food substance. Why, then, should the guinea pig suffer scurvy when restricted to a diet of oats and milk?

McCollum and Pitz found in the guinea pigs which had died of scurvy, that the cecum which is a very large and very delicate pouch through which the food must pass in going from the small to the large intestine, was always packed with putrefying feces.[16] They decided that the mechanical difficulty which the animals have in the removal of feces of an unfavorable character from this part of the digestive tract was in some way related with the development of the disease. That this assumption was correct, was shown by the fact that the administration of liquid petrolatum, a "mineral" product to which no food value can possibly be attributed, served to relieve a certain number of animals after they were near death from the disease, while confined strictly to the diet of oats and milk which caused them to develop scurvy. The explanation which they offered was that the liquid petrolatum served to improve the physical properties of the contents of the packed cecum, and thus enable the animals to rid themselves of this mass which was undergoing putrefactive decomposition.

Further experiments showed that when the animals were fed an oat and milk diet, to which was added suitable doses of phenolphthalein, a cathartic, they could withstand the diet for long periods without developing scurvy. This, according to McCollum and Pitz, was due to the additional secretion of water into the digestive tract, brought about by the cathartic, and resulted in softening the feces so that they were more easily eliminated from the cecum.

It has long been known that orange juice is a very efficient protective agent against scurvy, both in man and the guinea pig. In fact it was because of the spectacular relief of the disease by the administration of orange juice or of fresh vegetables, that Funk was led to the belief that scurvy is, like beri-beri, due to the lack of some specific chemical substance from the food supply. McCollum and Pitz further tested their theory by preparing an artificial orange juice, in which every constituent was known, and the administration of this to guinea pigs which were confined to a diet of oats and milk, on which food supply they almost invariably develop the disease. The "artificial orange juice" consisted only of citric acid, cane sugar and inorganic salts, in about the proportions in which these occur in the edible portion of the orange. It was demonstrated that this mixture exerted a decidedly protective action when added to the oat and milk diet, and prevented the development of scurvy over a long period.

Jackson and Moore suggested that scurvy is a bacterial disease, and they have secured experimental evidence which strongly supports that view. They found in the hemorrhagic joints a diploccocus, which may have a causal relationship to the disease. They

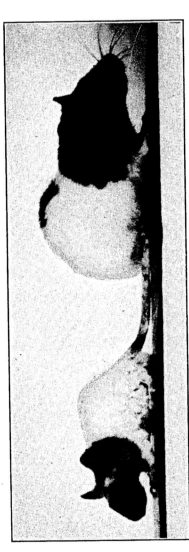

Fig. 9.—The rations of these two rats had the same composition as shown by chemical analysis. They differed only in the source of the protein which they contained. The rat on the right grew up on a mixture of proteins from the corn kernel and wheat gluten; that on the left on a mixture of corn proteins and gelatin. The difference in size, and remarkable difference in appearance is solely the result of the difference in the quality of the proteins in the two diets. Corn proteins and gelatin do not supplement each other's amino-acid deficiencies. (See legend to Chart 8. Lots 651 and 649.)

were able to induce mild symptoms of scurvy by the injection of bacterial cultures into animals which were fed upon a diet which regularly maintains the guinea pig in a state of health. McCollum and Pitz hold the view that there may be an invasion of the tissues by organisms as the result of injury to the cecal wall, when the animals are debilitated. The cecum is injured by long contact with the irritating products formed by putrefactive bacteria acting on the protein substances contained in the cecum when it becomes packed with feces of such a character that they cannot be eliminated. They suggested the alternative hypothesis that there may be formed through bacterial activity, substances which are toxic, and have such pharmacological properties as cause injury to the walls of the capillaries of those areas in which hemorrhage is observed in scurvy. There are several problems still to be solved in connection with the cause of scurvy, but it seems to be satisfactorily demonstrated that it is not a "deficiency" disease in the sense in which are beri-beri and the type of xerophthalmia of dietary orgin. There is, according to McCollum and his co-workers, no protective substance against this disease. Diets of faulty character, and especially bacteriologically unsatisfactory, are responsible for its etiology, and it is relieved by a satisfactory diet. The peculiar anatomical structure of the alimentary tract of the guinea pig makes it difficult for it to thrive unless its diet contains a succulent vegetable, which gives the feces favorable physical characters and which makes them easy of elimination.

Hess [17] has recently described the results of his observations on infants which were fed milk treated in various ways, and these are of great significance in throwing light on the cause of scurvy. He points out that for a period of two years milk which had been pasteurized commercially at 165° for thirty minutes was employed in feeding the infants in his charge. For two subsequent years the dealers raised it to only 145° for thirty minutes. In his experience the former milk was more likely to induce scurvy than the latter. Hess thereafter secured raw certified milk and pasteurized it at the institution for thirty minutes at 145.° Infants fed this milk did not develop scurvy in any instance, and one which showed symptoms of subacute scurvy improved on the home pasteurized milk. How did this milk differ from the commercially pasteurized milk which did show definite tendency to induce the disease? He points out that it differed mainly in the interval which elapsed between the time of the heating process and the time of consumption of the milk. In New York City, the greater portion of the bottled milk sold is of Grade B, most of which is brought to the city for pasteurization, which is done soon after midnight. Much of this is delivered to the consumer the following morning, but a part is allowed to stand until the following day before delivery. The city milk of Grade A was largely pasteurized in the country, and since they stored the milk for twenty-four hours after the heat treatment so as to insure a constant supply in case of delay in the delivery from the country, there was an interval of forty-eight hours between the pasteurization and the delivery of the milk to the consumer. Hess reproduced these conditions in his institution by keeping milk pasteurized at 145° for forty-eight hours on ice. Of eight infants which were fed the milk so treated, two showed scorbutic symptoms, which were relieved by giving them orange juice. Two out of another eight which were fed milk which was kept on ice forty-eight hours after the heat treatment showed signs of scurvy. In other cases scurvy was observed in infants fed certified milk which had not been pasteurized, when the latter had been kept on the ice forty-eight hours before feeding. Ageing is, therefore, effective in causing changes in both raw and pasteurized milk, so that the danger of the development of scurvy in infants to which it is fed is increased.

Boiled milk has been extensively fed to infants in various parts of the world and in the experience of some observers does not induce scurvy. The experience of Hess further supports the view that boiled milk is less liable to induce scurvy than is milk which has been pasteurized at 165° or at a lower temperature. Milk which has been pasteurized at 165° is more liable to induce scurvy than either boiled milk, or milk which has been pasteurized at lower temperatures, as 140–145° for thirty minutes. The most satisfactory explanation for these results seems to be found in the bacteriological condition of the milks treated in the various ways described. Heating milk at 165° kills nearly all the lactic acid forming bacteria which normally cause the souring of milk. Heating for thirty minutes at 140° to 145° leaves some of the organisms capable of development, and milk so pasteurized will sour. In the absence of the acid formers there develop during the interval between heating and consumption the spore-forming organisms which are not killed by pasteurization. These will, in time, cause the putrefactive decomposition of the milk. Any heat treatment which kills all the acid formers leaves the milk in a suitable condition for the development of the pernicious forms, and old milk so treated may be a menace to the health of infants, and unfit for consumption by adults. Boiling tends to destroy all the organisms in milk and will do so if sufficiently prolonged. Such milk may be more suitable for food than that which has been so treated as to prevent souring and yet be in a condition to permit the growth of putrefactive forms of bacteria. These results strongly support the view that there is a bacteriological factor involved in the causation of scurvy, and emphasizes the importance of securing clean milk, and of having it so handled as to insure its delivery in a good bacteriological condition. Milk should not be kept in the home without efficient refrigeration, and should be consumed before it becomes stale. Pasteurization seems, in itself, to

have little influence in lowering the food value of
milk. The staleness is the great element of danger.
Pasteurization is desirable as a safeguard against
such diseases as typhoid fever, tuberculosis, scarlet
fever and such organisms as cause epidemics of sore
throat. It does not render milk permanently harmless. The public should insist upon having its milk
supply produced under hygienic conditions. Milk
should then be cooled promptly so as to depress as
far as possible the growth of the organisms which
always find entrance through the air and from the
cow and the milker. It should be carefully refriger-
ated, and promptly delivered and properly cared for
in the home, and should not be allowed to age un-
necessarily before use. If pasteurized, it should pref-
erably receive the lowest heat treatment which will
effectively destroy the pathogenic organisms, and
should be delivered as promptly as possible thereafter in a suitably cooled state. Stale milk is danger-
ous, especially for use in infant feeding.

Pellagra.—This disease has been common in parts
of Europe for centuries. It is especially common in
northern Italy, and has been sometimes referred to
as Alpine scurvy. It is likewise known in Spain and
and the south of France. The disease was first observed in America in 1907, and has been steadily
on the increase, especially in certain of the Southern
States. In 1917 it was estimated that there were
165,000 pellagrins in the United States.

Pellagra is essentially a disease of poverty, although there are many cases recorded among the well-to-do. It has been especially prevalent in the country, in villages, and in the poorer sections of cities, and is observed to occur most frequently following periods of scarcity of food. In Europe the disease was long associated with the consumption of spoiled maize as the chief article of diet, but it is now known that the eating of this grain has nothing whatever to do with its causation. All observers are agreed that the diet is of primary import in the etiology of the disease, but differences of opinion still exist as to whether there is likewise a bacteriological factor involved.

The trouble begins with digestive disturbances of an indefinite character, followed by soreness of the mouth, which renders eating difficult, and a persistent diarrhea which saps the strength of the patient. Skin eruptions appear, and there are formed on parts of the body dark crusts which sometimes suppurate. In severe cases there are pronounced nervous disturbances preceding death.

In its early stages pellagra yields fairly readily to dietetic treatment. Indeed it has been emphasized by clinicians that without dietary measures, there is no effective treatment, and numerous cases are recorded in which the disease has disappeared promptly when milk, eggs and meats, string beans, together with a liberal amount of the leafy vegetables, such as cabbage, collards, and lettuce, were included in the diet.[18]

In the United States, especially, pellagra tends to seasonal occurrence, most new cases occurring in the spring, or better, as Goldberger has emphasized, at the end of winter. Jobling, in his excellent survey of pellagra in Nashville, found that nearly all cases had their onset in the spring and early summer.[19] It frequently happens that sufferers recover from their attacks of the disease during the later summer and fall, and suffer a relaspe during the following spring. Indeed the diet of many of the poorer people of the South, during the winter, consists principally of corn bread, pork and molasses. From what has been said in earlier chapters, it will be easily appreciated that such a combination of food-stuffs does not constitute an adequate diet, and it is significant that nearly all new cases develop after a hundred days or more of confinement to such a food supply.

It should be pointed out that Jobling and Peterson emphasize that from their observations the pellagrins, and the class from which the new cases develop, consume relatively much carbohydrate and relatively little protein, since they make liberal use of corn bread, corn grits, and potatoes and biscuits made from bolted flour, together with molasses, There were some who declared that they had regularly eaten eggs, butter milk, milk and meat. They further point out that in the spring, summer and autumn months a great deal of green stuff in the form of turnip tops, wild mustard, green peas (seed) and green onions are eaten. The green onions are eaten raw, the others cooked. In addition, during the summer months much fruit, especially peaches and apples, are eaten since these are usually cheap. In commenting upon the studies of Goldberger, Jobling and Peterson point out that the poorly nourished individual is prone to contract many diseases and their observation that there is a close relationship between the sanitary condition of the different parts of Nashville and the incidence of pellagra, tends to strongly support the view that the disease is associated with poor sewage disposal. The sanitary conditions in those districts where pellagra is common are of the worst sort, in many instances there being little pretense made of doing anything with the excreta, which during the summer is usually covered with flies. Screening was usually absent from those houses where the disease was found. Jobling and Peterson are essentially in accord with the conclusions of the Thompson-McFadden Commission [20] which made a thorough investigation of conditions in Spartanburg County, S. C., where pellagra is a scourge, and arrived at the conclusion that the disease is in some way related to a bacteriological factor, and is probably distributed by an insect.

Golderger has accomplished a great work in demonstrating that the diet, when properly constituted, causes the disappearance of pellagra, and prevents its recurrence. His dietary studies have demonstrated beyond a reasonable doubt that a faulty diet is the most important factor in causing the development of the condition. He has shown that when liberal amounts of milk and eggs and of meat, are introduced into the diet of institutions, such as insane asylums and orphanages, in which the disease was previously common, they become free from it even though new cases are admitted freely and the sick are mingled with the well. He and his co-workers have likewise made heroic attempts to transmit the disease to themselves by means of the administration of the excreta and material from the lesions of pellagrins, but without success, when the experimenters were taking a satisfactory diet.[21]

An experiment on man, which was carried out by Goldberger, is of special interest. A diet consisting of dishes prepared from degerminated corn meal, bolted wheat flour, rice, starch, sugar, pork fat, together with sweet potatoes, cabbage, collards, turnip greens and coffee, induced the appearance of what were regarded as the incipient signs of the disease by the end of five and a half months in five of eleven men, who volunteered to submit themselves to this dietary régime.[22]

Chittenden and Underhill[23] have described experiments in which dogs were restricted to a diet of crackers (wheat flour), cooked (dried) peas and cottonseed oil. After intervals varying from two to eight months, the animals developed the typical sore mouth, severe diarrhea and skin changes strikingly suggestive of pellagra in man. They were of the opinion that this diet caused these symptoms because of the lack of some substance or substances of the class designated as "vitamines" by Funk.

McCollum, Simmonds and Parsons [24] demonstrated that the diet of Chittenden and Underhill, which consisted of bolted wheat flour, peas and cottonseed oil, cannot be deficient in any other unidentified dietary essential than the fat-soluble A, a lack of which is associated with the development of the eye disease, xerophthalmia. This conclusion is necessary since rats were shown to fail to grow or remain in a state of health, on this mixture, and that it is rendered dietetically sufficiently complete by the addition of three types of purified food substances, viz., mineral salts, protein, and fat-soluble A, to induce growth at the normal rate. The animals failed, however, to successfully rear young. The first limiting factor is the inorganic content. Everything of an unknown chemical nature which the diet must contain is present in a mixture of wheat flour, peas and cottonseed oil, but there is a relative shortage of the fat-soluble A, which is abundant in certain fats, and is associated with cellular structures generally in both animal and vegetable food-stuffs. McCollum, Simmonds and Parsons pointed out that although their rats failed to maintain satisfactory nutrition on this food mixture, unless the three kinds of supplements were added, there was no soreness of the mouth or diarrhea, such as was observed by Chittenden and Underhill in dogs, and are usually present in pellagra in man. The eyes became swollen when the diet was supplemented only by salts.

An inspection of the diets described by Goldberger as common in those institutions where pellagra is prevalent, and the winter diets of people in those districts where there is a high incidence of the disease in the spring and summer months, shows that these are composed largely of seeds and seed products, and the amounts of leafy vegetables, milk, eggs and meat, are very small, or are entirely absent, for varying periods. McCollum and Simmonds [25] have pointed out that in the experimental diet with which Goldberger reported having produced incipient pellagra in man, about ninety-six per cent of the total solids of the food supply was derived from seed products: corn meal, wheat flour, rice, starch, sugar, molasses and from pork fat, and only about four per cent from sweet potatoes and the leafy vegetables together. Such a small amount of the leaf does not suffice to make good the dietary deficiencies of the seed products in such a diet. These deficiencies are now well understood, and it is further known that the tubers, such as the potato and sweet potato, are not so constituted as to serve as "protective" foods when taken together with seed products. The diets of those people who suffer from pellagra are, therefore deficient in three respects. They are relatively low in protein and their proteins are of relatively poor biological value, because they do not yield on digestion, a favorable mixture of amino-acids for the transformation into body tissues. They lack a sufficient amount of the unidentified dietary essential fat-soluble A, and also of certain mineral elements. The latter fault is in most instances limited to a shortage of calcium, sodium and chlorine. Since it is the regular practice of man to make additions of sodium chloride in the form of table salt, to his diet, the mineral deficiency in these diets may be said to be limited to the element calcium. Any one of these faults alone is sufficient to induce malnutrition when either the young or the adult animal is restricted to such diets as are common in pellagra stricken districts.

Since, however, there seems to be good evidence that there sometimes occur cases of pellagra in individuals whose diets have included a certain amount of such articles as McCollum and his co-workers have designated as PROTECTIVE FOODS, viz., milk, eggs and the leafy vegetables, the theory of an infection is supported. The prevalence of the disease in badly sewered districts supports this view. That there is a bacteriological factor involved in pellagra is further supported in some degree by the fact that McCollum, Simmonds and Parsons [25] observed only malnutrition without diarrhea or sore mouth in rats fed diets which in the experience of Chittenden and Underhill produce in dogs the gastro-intestinal symptoms seen in pellagra in man. The sloughing of the mucous membranes of the mouth, and the presence of ulcers in the intestine affords conclusive evidence of an infection in their dogs. McCollum and co-workers found no unhealthy appearance in the mucosa of the digestive tract, even when their rats were moribund as the result of being fed only wheat flour, peas and cottonseed oil. It seems probable that the difference in this respect in the two species may well be attributed to a chance infection in the one case which did not occur in the other. These observations are in harmony with the fact that not everyone who takes the poor diets described develops the disease. It seems logical in the light of all the data available, to conclude that poor nutrition predisposes to infection, and that there is an infectious agent involved in the production of pellagra. There can be no reasonable doubt that the possibility that pellagra is a "deficiency" disease, in the sense in which Funk employed this term, is definitely answered in the negative by the experimental work of McCollum and his co-workers.

Rickets.—There can be no doubt that rickets is a nutritional disease, but its relation to the diet is not clear. It is characterized especially by an alteration in the growth of the bones. These become enlarged at the extremities and so soft that they bend under the stress of muscular contraction and under the weight of the body. It is a disease of the first two years of life, and is especially prevalent in children in whose diet milk is replaced too largely by cereals and other vegetable foods, not suited to the delicate digestive tract of the young child. Predisposing factors in many cases are undoubtedly tuberculosis and syphilis. The symptoms develop gradually. Restlessness and perspiration at night, great sensitiveness of the limbs, that even a light touch is extremely painful, are characteristic signs of the disease. There are gastro-intestinal disturbances, especially colic and distension of the intestine with gas, so that the abdomen protrudes. The bones become thickened, and nodules develop at the junctures of the ribs with the costal cartilages, forming the characteristic "beaded" ribs. There is defective ossification of the skull; the teeth appear later than normal and in unusual order. Various deformities of the head, spine, chest and limbs result as the child develops. Recovery with deformity is of frequent occurrence.

There must, at the present time, be an element of speculation in any discussion of the relation of diet to rickets. The well-known deficiencies from the dietary standpoint of the cereal grains and the other storage organs, together with the injury to the intestine, which is nearly always present, as shown by the distended abdomen, and the occurrence of rickets only in early life, and so frequently in association with infectious disease, all make it unnecessary to invoke the aid of any hypothetical "vitamine," to a lack of which the disease may be attributed.

Hess [26] has recently described the results of his dietary studies among the negro women of the Columbus Hill district in New York, whose children

almost all suffer from rickets. It is significant that
these women are attempting, like the very poor in
many cities, to live on a diet derived from the endosperm of wheat, maize and rice, bolted flour,
degerminated cornmeal, polished rice, together with
tubers and meats. It will be evident from the data
furnished by the application of the biological method
for the analysis of food-stuffs, which McCollum and
his co-workers have perfected, and which was described in Chapters I to III, that there are no combinations of those food-stuffs whose functions are
those of storage organs, which will constitute a satisfactory diet for growth. Muscle tissue does not tend,
except in respect to the protein factor, to correct the
dietary faults of such mixtures. The regular consumption of such diets will in the course of a few
months cause a distinct lowering of the vitality of
an adult and will cause even greater injury to the
young child. In a later chapter it will be shown that
the milk of mothers taking such diets does not
satisfactorily nourish the young.

What has said/been above regarding the special
dietary properties of the different food-stuffs which
go to make up the diet of civilized man, and the
dietary habits of those classes of people who suffer
from the diseases which have come to be recognized
as being due to faulty diet, make it easy to see that
there has become fixed in the minds of students of
nutrition and of the reading public, an altogether
extravagant idea regarding the importance of the

substances to which Funk gave the name "vitamines." Of the diseases which Funk considered due
to lack of unidentified substances of this nature,
viz., beri-beri, scurvy, pellagra and rickets, but one,
beri-beri, has been shown to be due to this cause.
In the course of the analysis by McCollum and Davis,
of the problem of what chemical complexes are necessary to constitute the simplest diet which will
serve to support growth in the young, and maintain
physiological well-being in the adult, a second dietary
"deficiency" disease in the same sense as beri-beri,
was discovered, and shown to have occurred sporad-
ically in man. This is the type of xerophthalmia
which results from a deficiency of the dietary essential of unknown chemical nature, fat-soluble A.
Beri-beri is due to the lack of the second unknown
dietary essential water-soluble B. Pellagra, scurvy
and rickets do not belong in the same category with
beri-beri, and there do not exist "curative" substances of unknown nature for these diseases. The
individual is predisposed to the development of these
syndromes by faulty diet, but the faults have been
shown by the biological method for the analysis of
the individual food-stuffs or their mixtures, to reside
in maladjustments, and unsatisfactory quantitative
relationships among the now well-recognized constituents of the normal diet. They are to be sought
in the quality and quantity of the protein, the character and amount of the inorganic constituents, the
physical properties of the residues which are left

after digestion, and form the feces from which the intestine must rid itself. It seems probable that the only unidentified substance which is physiologically indispensable, which is not sufficiently abundant in the diets employed by the people of the United States and Europe where there are used insufficient amounts of milk, butter, cream, eggs and the leafy vegetables, is the fat-soluble A, but occasionally diets may be met with which contain too little of the water-soluble B. Sufficient knowledge is now available to make it possible to select such foods as will mutually make good each other's deficiencies, and to combine them in such proportions as will insure the disappearance of all the diseases of man which are brought on by faulty diets. The same knowledge will, in the future, make possible an efficient utilization of feeding-stuffs for animal production, which will be of inestimable economic value to mankind.

CHAPTER VI

THE NURSING MOTHER AS A FACTOR OF SAFETY IN THE NUTRITION OF THE SUCKLING

Anyone who reflects upon the relation of the mother to her young during the suckling period, must marvel at the fact that during early life the young mammal cannot thrive on the diet of the adult. It must have milk for a shorter or longer period after birth. This the lactating animal is able to form from her food through the agency of the mammary gland. The period of dependency varies greatly in different species. Among mammals, with which the author is familiar, the young guinea pig is born in the most highly developed state. The newborn cavy is capable of eating grass or succulent vegetables during the first or second day of post-natal life. The young rat may be safely weaned at the age of twenty-five days, provided a highly satisfactory diet of the type which suffices for the adult is then supplied. The young pig (swine) becomes able to eat fairly liberally of the normal adult diet at the age of six or eight weeks, whereas the human infant must live largely on a milk diet during the first year of life and should have a liberal allowance of milk and of eggs during the entire growing period.

116

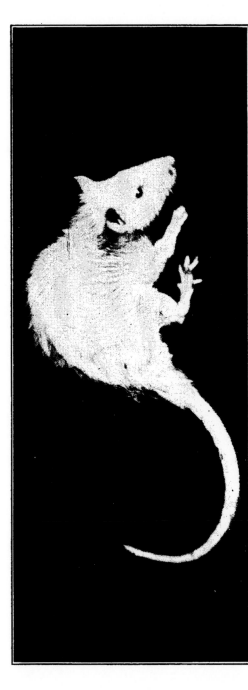

FIG. 10.—This picture illustrates the emaciated appearance of a middle aged rat after being fed about four months on a diet consisting of bolted flour, degerminated corn meal, rice, sugar, starch, pork fat, molasses, sweet potato, and cabbage. Such a diet has been reported by Goldberger to have produced pellagra in man in five and a half months. This diet affords wide variety and consists of wholesome food products, yet fails to maintain normal nutrition because it contains too little of the *protective foods*, milk, eggs and the leafy vegetables.

Even eggs will not entirely replace milk during any part of this period. It is of great importance that we should understand the relationship between the character of the diet of the lactating female, and the quality of the milk which she is able to produce. Our knowledge of this subject is still very incomplete, but experimental studies on animals have recently thrown light on certain very important phases of this problem.

In order to gain information on the relation between the character of the diet of the mother and the value of the milk which she produces, McCollum and Simmonds [1] carried out a series of experiments on lactating rats, whose diets were faulty in known ways, and observed the effect on the growth of the young which these mothers nursed. The mothers were fed a highly satisfactory diet until they had completed their term of pregnancy. As soon as the young were born, the litter was in all cases reduced to four, in order that the nutritive undertaking of the mother should in no case be burdensome. The mother was at once restricted to a diet which would not induce any growth whatever in a young rat after separation from the mother at weaning time. The diets of the mothers in the various experiments were faulty in respect to each of the factors which are necessary for the formation of a satisfactory diet, but the number of characters in which a single diet was faulty varied from one to three.

In one case the mother was fed upon a diet of

purified protein, carbohydrate (dextrinized starch), a suitably constituted inorganic salt mixture, and an alcoholic extract of wheat germ to furnish the unidentified dietary essential, water-soluble B. This diet contained everything necessary for the nutrition of a young rat during growth, except the fat-soluble A. The problem was to find whether the mother could, through the agency of the mammary gland, form the missing substance, fat-soluble A. Experience has shown that the young animal after the weaning age, cannot produce it *de novo*, for its own preservation from any of the other constituents of its food. The results of the experiment indicated that the quantity of the fat-soluble A in the milk produced from such a diet is below the amount necessary for the promotion of the maximum rate of growth in the young. It has been shown by Osborne and Mendel,[2] that the body fats of beef cattle contain a small amount of the fat-soluble A. It seems certain that the body fats of an animal which has been fed for some time on a diet rich in this substance, will serve as a reserve supply of this dietary essential, which the mother can secrete into the milk. In other experiments, Chart 15, definite evidence is presented that this substance is not abundant in the milk unless it is present in the diet of the mother. The presence of some fat-soluble A in the tissues of the mother makes it especially difficult to obtain milk which is entirely free from this s bstance.

Through similar experiments with diets which contained the fat-soluble A, but not the water-soluble B, evidence was secured that for a time the mother is able to secure this dietary factor from her reserve supply, but none of the growth curves indicated that the substance is present in the milk in adequate amount when the diet of the mother lacks it. It seems certain that neither of these substances is present in abundance in the milk of the mother, unless it is furnished in her food.

Evidence confirmatory of this view is found in the studies of Andrews [3] on infantile beri-beri. It is well known that the faulty diet of rice and fish, which furnishes the principal food of many of the poorer classes of the Orient, does not prevent the onset of beri-beri, and infants who nurse mothers who are suffering from the disease, likewise develop beri-beri. Andrews induced several Filipino women whose infants had just died of beri-beri, to nurse young pups, and noted that in all cases the latter failed to grow, became edematous, and lost the use of their hind legs. Paralysis of the posterior extremities is one of the symptoms of the disease in man. It is evident that in the milk of these mothers there was a shortage of the water-soluble B, for it is a shortage of this substance which causes the development of this syndrome.

It has been pointed out that young animals do not grow when confined to a single seed or mixture of seeds of plants, for the reason that these are all

lacking in sufficient amounts of the inorganic elements, calcium, sodium and chlorine, and are too
poor in the fat-soluble A to support normal nutrition.
The quality of their proteins is likewise too poor
to make them very satisfactory for the support of
growth. McCollum and Simmonds have studied
the extent to which the mother is able to produce
milk of satisfactory character for the promotion of
growth in the young, when confined to a single seed as
the sole source of nutriment. Charts 15 and 16 show
the effects of such diets on the growth of the young.

The curves of rat 211 and of her litter of four
young (Chart 15) illustrate the remarkable growth
which a mother rat is able to induce in her young
when her diet is highly satisfactory, and while
doing so, she is able to increase her own weight very
appreciably. In marked contrast to this "normal"
accomplishment stands the failure of rat 738 to induce more than one-third the normal rate of growth
in her young when restricted to rolled oats as her
sole food supply. The drop in the curve of the
young at the 40th day was the result of the death
of the young at brief intervals. The mother lost
weight regularly, showing that she was sacrificing
her own tissues for the preservation of her young.
Rolled oats, like the other seeds, require improvement in respect to three dietary factors before it
becomes a complete food, and on such a faulty diet
the mother produces milk which is not satisfactory
for the promotion of growth in her offspring.

Rat 843, whose diet consisted of rolled oats supplemented with fat-soluble A (as butter fat) induced growth in her young at a somewhat greater rate than she could have done, had she eaten oats alone, and was able to keep them alive for a longer period. The first one died on the 57th day and the others followed in rapid succession. This mother lost considerable weight up to the time that the young began to eat of the oat and butter fat diet. Young rats, after removal from the mother, cannot grow at all on this diet.

Rat 899, was fed a diet of rolled oats to which was added such an inorganic salt mixture as made good the mineral deficiencies of the oat kernel. Her diet was still deficient in fat-soluble A, and to some extent in the quality of its proteins. With this food her milk was of distinctly better quality than that which can be produced on a diet of oats alone, or on oats supplemented with fat-soluble A, or on oats supplemented with purified protein (rat 948). From these results it is apparent that the first limiting factor of the oat kernel for milk production in the lactating animal is the same as in the young for growth, viz., the inorganic content of the food supply.

The importance of having the inorganic content of the diet properly constituted is shown especially well in the performance of the mothers 983 and 1978. The former was fed rolled oats supplemented with both fat-soluble A, in the form of butter fat, and purified protein in the form of casein of milk.

Even with these two additions she was able to induce less than half normal growth in her young and they began to die at the age of 45 days, and all succumbed in rapid succession. Rat 1978, on the other hand, whose diet consisted of rolled oats supplemented with a suitable salt mixture and butter fat, was able to induce growth in her young at about two-thirds the normal rate. The improvement of the milk by the inclusion of fat-soluble A in the diet is very apparent, since the young did not die during the period of sixty days covered by the experiment, and supports the view that this substance cannot be synthesized by the mother.

Rat 1019, whose diet consisted of rolled oats supplemented with purified protein and a suitable salt mixture, shows that the mother is able to induce nearly the optimum rate of growth in her young during a period of thirty days, although her diet was very poor in the factor fat-soluble A. It should be borne in mind that the seeds, because they contain a small proportion of cellular structures in addition to their reserve food package in the endosperm, contain a small but inadequate amount of the fat-soluble A. The mother is able, when the diet of oats is corrected with respect to two factors, protein and salts, to concentrate in the milk the small content of the fat-soluble A which her diet supplies. She is probably also able to draw in some degree upon her small store of this substance which is deposited in her body fats, and supply the young with enough of it to

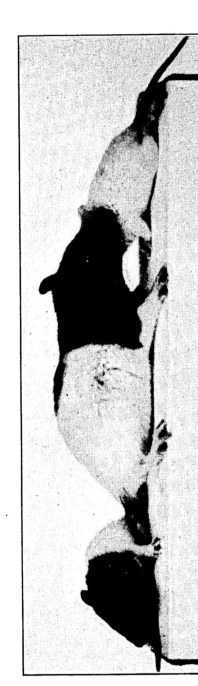

FIG. 11.—This illustration shows the great differences in the size, stage of development and vigor in young rats, which may result from faults in the character of the diets of the mothers which they are nursing. These three rats were the same age. The mother of the two little ones received a diet which was deficient in the quantity and quality of its proteins.

enable them to reach a state of relative independence, which in a wild state would enable them to go in search of food for themselves. There is abundant experimental proof that when the protein and inorganic content of the food are of highly satisfactory character, animals can subsist for a long period on a supply of fat-soluble A too small to prevent the onset of xerophthalmia in diets of lower biological value.

These records of nursing mothers and their young make it apparent that the former is limited in a general way in the utilization of food for milk production, in the same manner as in the growing young in the utilization of food for the construction of new body tissues. She is, however, a factor of safety for her young in no small degree. It should be remembered that a young rat cannot grow at all when, after the weaning age, it is limited to the oat kernel, or to the oat kernel supplemented with either salts, protein or fat-soluble A alone, or on a diet of oats supplemented with both protein and fat-soluble A. In order that it may grow even very slowly it is essential that both a suitable salt mixture and fat-soluble A shall be added to the oat kernel. It cannot grow normally unless the protein factor is likewise improved. In the records of the mothers and young shown in Chart 15, the young continued to grow in certain instances after the twenty-fifth day, the age at which they may be safely weaned when their milk supply has been of normal composition. This fact is conclusive evidence that even after the

young become able to eat of the diet on which the
mother had produced the milk on which they were
able to grow—a diet on which they would be unable
to grow at all without some corrections and improve-
ments—they were still receiving a supplementary
milk supply from the mother. This served to correct
in some measure the faulty diet of oats plus an incomplete supplementary addition. It seems certain
that milk production must have been very considerable in amount, to thus enhance the diet of
four young whose weight collectively was about half
that of the mother herself.

The inorganic content of all the seeds is the first
limiting factor in preventing growth in young animals, and in determining the quality of the milk which
can be produced from them. The young animal
cannot grow at all on seeds unless one of the factors
corrected includes certain salt additions, yet the
mother is able to produce milk without any such
additions, which is capable of inducing a limited
amount of growth in the young. It is apparent that
one of her most important relations to her helpless
offspring is her capacity to supply it with a better
inorganic food supply than she herself secures in her
food, when the latter is of poor quality.

The growth curves of the young of mothers whose
diets consisted of the oat kernel without and with
purified food additions, illustrate likewise very well
the results which are observed when similar experiments are conducted with the wheat or maize

kernel. They emphasize the fact that for milk production as for growth, the seeds of plants may be regarded as closely similar in their dietary properties. It is therefore, rendered highly probable that the same analogy runs through the series of food-stuffs in their value for the production of milk of normal character. We are not to expect, therefore, that a diet consisting of even a complex mixture of seeds, tubers and roots, will produce milk of highly satisfactory character, and without undue strain on the mother. It has been emphasized that even this list of foods of the class whose functions are those of storage organs, do not suffice even when combined with meat, to induce satisfactory growth in the young. It follows as a logical conclusion, that a lactating mother will not be able to produce milk of a very satisfactory character when she is restricted to such food-stuffs. It should be reiterated that there are two classes of food-stuffs which are so constituted as to correct the deficiencies of seeds, tubers, roots and meat. These are milk and the leaves of plants and they should be used very liberally in the diet. Eggs are in some degree to be regarded as comparable to these, but eggs have not the favorable mineral content of the leaves and of milk, and this is one of the most important factors in which the storage organs of plants need supplementing.

The question will arise in the minds of many, as to whether the inability of the young to grow on the milk produced by mothers which were living upon an inadequate diet, was not the result of the failure of the mothers to produce enough milk rather than milk of abnormal composition. It has not been found possible to secure complete information as to the actual amount of milk which these rats secreted, but we have analogous data from domestic animals, which support the view that milk secretion remains fairly constant in the lactating animal even under very unfavorable conditions of nutrition.

Babcock [4] has described experiments in which he deprived cows of common salt during lactation, other than that which they secured in their regular ration, which was of a type suitable for the dairy cow. The keen appetite of the herbivora for salt is a matter of common knowledge. Deer which are very shy will risk any danger to secure salt at their accustomed licks or from salt springs. The periods of salt deprivation varied from two to fifteen months, and some of the animals actually died, and others were saved from death by the administration of salt. In no instance was there a notable decrease in the yield of milk by these cows up to a short time before they began to fail rapidly. Indeed the fat content of the milk of the cows receiving an inadequate salt supply was slightly higher than in the milk of the control group.

Eccles and Palmer [5] have conducted a very thorough experimental study of the influence of underfeeding of cows on milk production, and have studied its composition in cows whose rations were of suitable composition, but inadequate in amount. These results show that cows were able, during the early part of the lactation period, to maintain the milk flow undiminished for forty days, when receiving but 75 per cent enough food to meet her requirements. Under such conditions of nutrition there was no pronounced change in the composition of the milk. During the latter part of the lactation period there was some falling off in milk production as the result of under-feeding.

Ducaisne [6] in 1870, noted that during the siege of Paris, young and vigorous women were able to produce enough milk to maintain their infants, and in some cases to increase their weight when they were partially fasting. These observations, as well as those of Andrews on women whose infants had died of beri-beri,[3] all support the view that under conditions of faulty nutrition, it is the quality of the milk rather than the quantity which early suffers impairment. Dr. Manuel Roxas, of the College of Agriculture of the Philippine Islands, has informed the author in a private communication, that the infants' death rate among the natives is much higher in the breast-fed than among the bottle-fed children.

The occurrence of infantile beri-beri, rather than of death from starvation, further serves to demonstrate that it is milk of poor quality, rather than lack of sufficient amount of milk which is responsible for the high infant mortality in those parts of the world where the poorer classes live too largely on food-stuffs derived from products whose biological functions are those of storage organs, and meat.

The statement which one sees reiterated so frequently, that breast feeding of infants is superior to the best system of artificial feeding, needs to be qualified to some extent. There are, without question, in many parts of the world, large groups of people whose diets are of such a character that the quality of the milk produced by the lactating mother is not such as to make it a satisfactory food for their infants. It should be thoroughly appreciated that the human mother should have in her diet a liberal amount of milk in order to safeguard the health and well-being of her infant, and of leafy vegetables, which serve the two-fold function of a protective food and of greatly aiding intestinal elimination. That some mothers can induce a fair amount of growth in their infants while taking a faulty diet, cannot be denied, but that both mother and child suffer impairment as the result is beyond question. It is not enough that the diet shall furnish enough calories and enough protein, and shall afford variety and palatability. The peculiar dietary properties of the food-stuffs which enter into the diet are of paramount importance, and must be taken into consideration.

Attention should again be directed to the observations of Hess[7] that the diet of the negro women of the Columbus Hill district in New York, whose diets are derived almost exclusively from seed products,

tubers and meats, fail to nourish their infants satisfactorily as shown by the almost universal prevalence
of rickets among the latter. It is difficult for man
to correct the dietary deficiencies of these products
by the use of the leaves of plants as his sole protective
food, because of the limited capacity of his digestive
tract. Milk in *liberal amounts* should always be
included in the diet of the lactating mother.

CHAPTER VII

PRACTICAL CONSIDERATIONS WHICH SHOULD GUIDE IN THE PLANNING OF THE DIET

In the preceding chapters there were presented data, which have been obtained by biological methods, concerning the special dietary properties of the several classes of natural food-stuffs, which enter into the diets of man and animals. It is evident from the experiments described that a diet may furnish an abundance of protein and energy, and may be easy of digestion, and may furnish a wide variety and include several seeds or products derived from these, together with tubers, roots and meats, and may be highly acceptable to the human palate and yet fail utterly to support satisfactory nutrition. In the light of such facts, it becomes apparent that a chemical analysis of a food-stuff throws no light whatever upon certain aspects of its dietary properties. It is only by biological methods that we can arrive at principles which can serve as a safe guide as to the method of procedure by means of which safe diets can be planned. In the present chapter will be discussed a number of questions which always arise in the minds of those who wish to apply the new knowledge to the planning of a suitable dietary régime.

It should be understood that it is neither necessary or desirable that we should abandon the customary classification of food-stuffs on the basis of chemical composition. We must have a language of nutrition, and consider foods on the basis of their protein, carbohydrate, fat, water and mineral content, as we have always done. We should be familiar with the quota of energy available from the different types of foods. We must, however, take into consideration certain facts which have not hitherto been considered, and concerning which a chemical analysis gives no information.

One of the outstanding results of modern research in nutrition is the great difference in the biological values of the proteins from different sources. In a general way this is appreciated by all well informed teachers of the present day, but many are still in need of clearer distinctions regarding what data in the literature are capable of direct application to practical nutrition, and what are of such a nature that they cannot be so applied. No lack of appreciation is intended of data of the latter type, for they may have, and indeed frequently have a value of the first importance to the investigator in this field. As an example may be cited the laborious studies through which the amino-acids became known, and the data yielded by such method of analysis of the proteins as those of Fischer and of Van Slyke. Important as are these results in making possible further progress, they are not of such a character that they can be applied, as has been frequently attempted, in making deductions concerning comparative food values. It is, however, through such studies that we have arrived at a satisfactory working hypothesis concerning the nature of the proteins, and have become able to appreciate why the proteins have different values in nutrition. Our analytical methods do not make possible an approximately quantitative determination of more than a third of the total number of the digestion products of the proteins. An attempt to utilize the figures for the yield of this or that amino-acid by one or another of the proteins, as evidence of the comparative values of the proteins themselves, or of the food-stuffs from which they are derived, will lead to entirely fallacious deduction.

Such data as are tabulated in the literature for the yields of the different amino-acids, make the pea and bean proteins appear superior to those of the cereal grains. McCollum and Simmonds have reported a long series of experiments with diets so planned that they were adequate in all respects, and the protein content was derived entirely from a single seed. The amount of protein in the diet was varied so as to find in one series what was the lowest per cent of protein in the food mixture which would just maintain a grown rat over a period of several months without loss of body weight, and in another series, the minimum amount of protein was determined which would induce in the young, half normal and full normal rate of growth respectively. The data regarding the values of several of the more important seed proteins for maintenance are of great interest. Rats can be maintained in body weight on suitably constituted diets containing 4.5 per cent of oat protein, or of millet seed protein; on 6 per cent of maize, rice or wheat proteins; on about 8 per cent of flax-seed protein, whereas it requires about 11 to 12 per cent of the proteins of the pea or the bean to accomplish the same result.

Chemical analysis shows the proteins of the pea and bean to contain all the known amino-acids, and none of these are present in excessive or in minimal quantities, whereas the wheat and maize proteins yield excessive amounts of one of them in particular. Glutamic acid, one of the digestion products of proteins, is present in the proteins of the muscle tissues of animals, in the case of no less than half a dozen species, to the extent of twelve to fourteen per cent. The same acid is present in the two principal proteins of the wheat kernel to the extent of nearly 40 per cent, and in the principal protein of the maize kernel to the extent of about 25 per cent. These proteins show other differences in composition which led to the belief that they were of relatively low biological value for growth, before they were studied satisfactorily by appropriately planned feeding experiments, all of which have confirmed this view. The observation that the split pea and navy bean proteins are of much less value in nutrition came therefore as a distinct surprise, since these results were not what were expected, in view of the tabulated yields of the several amino-acids shown by the most careful chemical analysis. The data obtained by properly planned feeding experiments are highly reliable, those from the chemical analysis very unsafe, from which to draw deductions.

It should be understood that these values for the proteins of the seeds apply only to the proteins of the single seed when fed as the sole source of protein. When fed in mixtures of two or more proteins having individually low values for the support of growth, they may mutually make good each other's amino-acid deficiencies, and form a mixture which is better than either constituent when fed singly. Since this was to be expected, McCollum, Simmonds and Parsons have made many feeding trials with simple combinations of two seeds, such as two cereal grains, one cereal and one legume seed (pea, bean); one seed and one leaf, etc., as the sole source of protein in the diet, and have sought to find which are the most fortunate combinations of the most important food-stuffs for the production of protein mixtures of high biological values for the support of growth. These trials have shown that, while such mixtures of proteins are superior to the individual foods fed separately as sources of protein, it has not been found possible to obtain protein mixtures from vegetable sources which even approximate the value of milk proteins, for the support of maintenance or growth.

The nitrogen-containing compounds of the potato have been lauded by several investigators as being of extraordinary value as a source of protein. McCollum, Simmonds and Parsons have studied the proteins of the potato, both for maintenance and growth, in experiments in which this tuber served as the sole source of protein, and all its dietary deficiencies were made good by suitable additions of purified food substances. These all indicate that when fed as the sole source of protein, the nitrogen compounds of the potato have a distinctly lower value than have the proteins of the cereal grains, oat, wheat, rice and maize.

Enough has been said regarding the great differences in the values of the proteins from different sources, to make it clear that it is impossible to say how much protein the diet should contain without having a knowledge of the values of the proteins which the diet contains. Chemical methods of analysis are not yet sufficiently perfected to throw any appreciable light on the values of the mixtures of proteins which occur in our natural foods.

The great attractiveness of the "vitamine" hypothesis of Funk, as an explanation for all the states of malnutrition which are referable to faulty diet, has led, in recent years, to much discussion of the question of the possible deterioration of foods during cooking, canning and drying. The demonstration by McCollum and his co-workers that there are but two unidentified dietary essentials, and but two dietary "deficiency" diseases, due respectively to a shortage of one or the other of these substances, fat-soluble A and water-soluble B, and that there are no "growth determinants" unnecessary for the maintenance of health in the adult, does not minimize the importance of this subject. The work of a number of investigators has shown that the water-soluble B, the protective substance against beri-beri, is readily destroyed when an excess of even such weak alkalies as soda are added to the food, suggests that this substance may be of an unstable character.

Osborne and Mendel [1] have shown that butter fat may have a blast of steam passed through it for two hours and still retain its peculiar growth-promoting properties, due to the presence of the fat-soluble A. This observation is in harmony with those of McCollum and Davis, that heating butter fat at the temperature of boiling water does not affect its peculiar dietary value. It is apparent, therefore, that any conditions to which milk fats are liable to be subjected during the cooking of foods will not greatly alter its value as a source of the fat-soluble A. McCollum and Simmonds have recently (unpublished data) tested a sample of butter fat prepared from evaporated milk, furnished to them by Dr. Lucius P. Brown of New York City, and have found it very effective in relieving the xerophthalmia in rats, brought on by the lack of the fat-soluble A in their diets. It appears, therefore, that there is no great deterioration in the quality of milk fats brought about by the processes of removal of water in the preparation of condensed or evaporated milks. They have likewise shown, as have also Osborne and Mendel, that dried milks still contain the fat-soluble A in abundance. There can be no serious objection to the use of dried or canned milks on the basis of their value with respect to this dietary essential.

The situation is likewise quite clear with respect to the ordinary dried foods. Leaves such as celery tops and those of the immature alfalfa plant, when dried in the ordinary way, are still good sources of the fat-soluble A. The alfalfa leaves were dried in the sun and the celery tops by artificial heat in a current of air after a preliminary treatment with steam.

McCollum and Davis [2] have pointed out that wheat germ can be moistened and heated in an autoclave at fifteen pounds pressure for an hour or more without any extensive destruction of the water-soluble B, and McCollum, Simmonds and Pitz [3] have subjected soaked navy beans to similar treatment without causing any great deterioration with respect to this dietary factor. This treatment is comparable to that to which fruits and vegetables are subjected when processed in canning, and shows that the widespread belief that canned foods have lost these dietary essentials is, at least, generally without foundation. The cooking of beans or greens with the addition of soda, which is a common practice, may cause the destruction of one or both of the unidentified dietary essentials. At least in the case of the water-soluble B, this will probably be true if sufficient soda is added to render the food alkaline. The use of soda in biscuit making will, according to Voegtlin, and Sullivan [4] cause the destruction of the water-soluble B, for they found that corn meal cooked with soda was no longer effective in causing the "cure" of beri-beri in pigeons.

In this connection it should be borne in mind that our ordinary foods all contain several times the amount of the water-soluble B which is necessary for the maintenance of growth and health in animals. There seems to be no valid reason why, if it is necessary for culinary purposes, to use soda in the cooking of a few foods, the practice should be discontinued. If the diet is so planned as to furnish a suitable quota of milk, and of cereals and other foods which are not so treated as to destroy the water-soluble B there is no danger of a shortage of this substance in the diet. *It is now well demonstrated that with the diets employed in Europe and America there is no such thing as a "vitamine" problem other than that of securing an adequate amount of the substance fat-soluble A.* Seeds and their products, tubers, roots and meats in the amount in which they are ordinarily consumed, do not furnish enough of this substance for the maintenance of an optimum state of well-being. Diets composed of these substances exclusively, may, when their other deficiencies are corrected, contain enough of the fat-soluble A to induce fairly good growth to nearly the full adult size, and may long prevent the development of xerophthalmia. They do not supply enough of it to support maximum vigor over a long period, and fall short of the amount necessary under the special conditions involved in pregnancy and lactation.

There is a wide-spread belief that wheat is superior to the other cereals as a food. There is no experimental evidence that this is true. Rye, barley, oats and maize resemble wheat very closely in their dietary properties, and it is safe to say that these can entirely replace wheat in the diet of children, adults and invalids without the least detriment to health. Those who have become accustomed to the use of wheat bread, are attached to it principally because of habit. Dietary habits become very firmly fixed and are hard to break away from. Millions in the Orient are greatly attached to rice as a food, and feel that they cannot live without it, whereas, we in America cannot bring ourselves to eat liberally of it in the simple and unappetizing form in which it is entirely acceptable in the Oriental. The Italian feels that no diet is satisfactory unless it contains macaroni. Garlic and other flavors which appeal to the appetite of certain peoples are disliked by others. These prejudices and many others are not expressions of physiological need, but are purely demands for something to which we have become accustomed. When properly cooked, cornmeal, oats and other cereals have never been shown to produce digestive disturbances. Reports that the people of Belgium, when restricted to the scanty fare which could be furnished them after the occupation of their territory by Germany, suffered from digestive disturbances from eating corn bread, are not to be taken as evidence that the corn products were in themselves responsible for the trouble. They were the sequel of an inadequate diet which impaired the vitality.

Experiments have been described, showing that bolted wheat flour is inferior to whole wheat.[5] If two pigeons are fed whole wheat and bolted flour respectively, while a third is allowed to fast, the first will remain in a state of apparent health for several weeks, the second will lose weight and die earlier than the fasting one. This does not mean that bolted flour is poisonous, but only that it is a more incomplete food than whole wheat. The pigeon which is fed whole wheat will succumb in the course of time, for whole wheat is not a complete food. The pigeon which fasts gradually wastes away, but slowly, because all the tissues decrease in volume and its physiological processes slow down. The bird which is fed the bolted flour dies earlier than the fasted one, because the burden of digesting and metabolizing a liberal intake of food requires that his metabolic processes go on at a rapid rate. When this demand is made upon it and its diet is so incomplete that there can be no repair of its wasted tissues, it wears out the more quickly. Such demonstrations do not constitute an argument against the use of wheat flour as a food. In so far as the latter supplies protein, energy and inorganic salts, it is a good food. What we should realize is that none of our vegetable foods or the meats are complete and ideal foods. Some are more deficient than others, and their deficiencies are not all alike. Satisfactory nutrition is to be attained only through the employment of the right combinations of foods, and in such proportions as will insure that the resulting diet will be properly constituted. We should accept our natural foods for what they are, and make proper use of them, rather than condemn this or that one because it is lacking in some respect.

It is fallacious reasoning to attempt to compare the money value of certain foods with certain others. We may safely compare the cost of the cereal grains or the legumes with each other, or with the tubers such as the potato or the sweet potato, or with the root foods. It is not possible to compare the cost of any of these with milk or the leafy vegetables such as cabbage, cauliflower, Swiss chard, collards, Brussel sprouts, onions, lettuce, celery tops, spinach, turnip tops and other leaves employed as greens. Milk and the leafy vegetables are to be regarded as *protective foods*. In some degree eggs are to be considered in the same class. Milk and the leafy vegetables should be taken in liberal amounts. The leaves should not be regarded as foods of low value because their content of protein, fat and carbohydrate is low, and the content of water high. When compared on the basis of chemical composition they appear inferior to seeds, but they have a peculiar value in their high content of fat-soluble A and of mineral elements, which makes them stand in a class by themselves among the vegetable food-stuffs.

No thorough studies of the dietary properties of fruits have yet been made, but from their known chemical composition and biological functions as storage organs, their proper place in the diet can be predicted. They are good sources of mineral salts and of energy-yielding foods, the sugars. They are highly palatable and exert a favorable influence on the excretory processes of the kidneys and the intestine. Their liberal use in the diet should be encouraged.

Owing to the present shortage of certain food-stuffs, there has been a tendency to consider the introduction of certain new products hitherto not generally employed in a large way as human foods, and to extend their use by extolling their virtues. Conspicuous among these are the peanut press cake, which remains after the oil is extracted by pressure, the soy bean and cottonseed flour. The latter product represents a portion of the cottonseed which is prepared by first removing the oil, and afterward grinding and bolting to obtain a product free from hulls and fiber. These movements directed toward the utilization of all our food resources are laudable, but the information which is disseminated concerning these products by their enthusiastic promoters is not in all cases accurate and sufficiently complete to serve as a safe guide to the user. They are extolled in the time-honored fashion as foods rich in protein and energy, but their exact place in the dietary is not sufficiently emphasized.

There can be no doubt that the peanut is a wholesome food, and can be used to advantage in the diet of man in moderate amounts. It is likewise a good source of protein of fairly good quality. The same can be said of the soy bean. The proteins of neither of these have extraordinary values. That there are no proteins of extraordinary values in the seeds of plants yet studied, is apparent from a critical and unprejudiced inspection of all of the extensive experimental data available. The point to be emphasized in this connection, is that *these are seed products, and have in a general way the peculiar dietary properties common to seeds.* Their place in the diet is therefore clear. They may be employed in moderate amounts along with other seeds and seed products, provided that they are supplemented with sufficient amounts of the *protective foods*, milk and the leafy vegetables.

With respect to cottonseed products the case is somewhat different. The cottonseed has long been known to contain something toxic to animals, and experience has taught that cottonseed meal, a product containing the hulls, cannot be fed liberally to animals without disastrous results. Withers and Carruth [6] have conducted extensive investigations regarding

the nature of the toxic constituent, and have isolated it as a substance to which the name gossypol
has been given. It is destroyed by oxidation, and
by appropriate heat treatment, and some cottonseed products are much less poisonous than others,
because of the special treatment which they have
received. The author has fed cottonseed flour to a
large number of animals, and is convinced that it
should not be employed in the human dietary in very
liberal amounts. If the diet is appropriately constituted with respect to its content of the protective
foods, cottonseed flour which has been thoroughly
cooked, will, when used in moderation, be found to be
a useful food-stuff. The data available emphasize the
need for further careful studies to show how much
heat treatment is necessary to render cottonseed
flour harmless. Such knowledge, when available,
will make possible the standardization of commercial
products, and will make possible the utilization of
this vast food resource.

The paramount importance of maintaining and
of increasing the production of milk makes it necessary to utilize a large amount of protein-rich foods in
the dairy industry. The wisest plan is to extend the
use of peanut, soy bean and cottonseed products for
milk production. The cow produces much of her
milk from coarse feeds, not suitable for human consumption, but requires liberal protein-rich supplements in addition. Greater emphasis should be laid
upon the wisdom of a more liberal purchase of milk

by the public. This would insure the best utilization of these protein-rich products which have not as yet in many quarters found extensive use as human foods. Experimental data seems to have established that the proteins of the peanut and the soy bean are of better quality than those of the pea or the navy bean. From the author's studies of the soy bean it appears that its proteins have about the same quality as those of the cereal grains, but it contains three times as much protein as the latter. Its content of fat-soluble A is such that a mixture of soy bean and starch which has the same protein content as the wheat kernel, probably has about the same dietary properties as has wheat with respect to these two dietary factors. There is no reason why the peanut and soy bean should not be employed to a greater extent as human foods, but it should be kept in mind that good use is already being made of these products in the feeding of dairy cows, and that if they are withdrawn from this application for use as human foods directly, it will not be easy to find something to take their place in the dairy industry.

Several writers have pointed out that these seeds contain the fat-soluble A, and have exhibited growth curves which indicate that animals have taken one of these seeds properly supplemented so as to correct its deficiencies, and have been able to grow to approximately the full adult size without the addition of more of this dietary essential. The reader is left with the impression that the peanut, soy bean and cottonseed may serve as an adequate source of fat-soluble A. This impression is an unfortunate one, for it is certain that even with diets which are composed largely of these seeds, the content of this substance is below the optimum, and in the amounts in which they are likely to enter into the human diet, they will never serve as a substitute for the protective foods. In the enthusiastic application of the biological method for the analysis of food-stuffs, by those with little experience, after its description by McCollum and Davis in 1915,[7] hasty conclusions have been drawn in a number of instances. McCollum and Simmonds have emphasized the necessity of observing over long periods, such animals as are able to grow at about the normal rate and produce a few young and rear them, when confined to experimental diets. In many instances it is found that the interval between litters is too long, or the mortality of the young abnormally high, the time necessary to bring the young to the weaning stage too long and the signs of old age appear too early, in animals which during the early part of the reproductive period appeared to be nearly normal in all respects. They have reached the conclusion that it is necessary to observe the behavior of the second generation when confined to the diet of the parent before drawing final conclusions concerning the quality of a diet. In many instances lack of vitality is first observed in the inability of the offspring to develop normally on a diet which would, in the early

life of the parent, have been considered entirely satisfactory. When observations are extended in this
way, it becomes apparent that lung infections very
frequently terminate the lives of the animals, whose
diets are faulty in some degree, but not so faulty as to
make their effects strikingly apparent.

From many questions asked by the public the author has gained the conviction that faulty deductions
have been drawn by others from experimental
studies, which would lead the inexperienced reader
to conclude that by the use of any seed products, or
other food-stuffs of vegetable origin, whose functions are those of storage organs, that diets can be
prepared which are so satisfactory as to make it
feasible to dispense with a liberal intake of the food-
stuffs which we have designated as *protective foods*.
These can be shown to be based upon failure to fully
appreciate what constitutes a satisfactory demonstration of the adequacy of a diet. Mankind will do
well to avoid such diets which may, as Golderger
has suggested, place one in "a 'twilight' zone within
which a very slight change in any of the dietary
components may cause an important shift of bal-
ance."

McCollum and Simmonds have reported many
experiments with diets so planned as to be satisfactory in that all the factors but one afforded a liberal
margin of safety in offering an abundance over the
minimal requirements of the animal,[8] and the remaining one so adjusted as to represent the actual

minimum on which the animal can subsist over a considerable period. In this way it has been possible to demonstrate that the amount of fat-soluble A may be reduced to a certain minimum without the development of xerophthalmia, whereas the same intake of this substance will not prevent the characteristic eye trouble when the intake of protein is likewise sufficiently lowered. They have been able to so adjust the components of the diet as to make it possible to relieve xerophthalmia either by increasing the content of protein or of fat-soluble A in the food, although it is the lack of the latter which is the specific cause of the disease. Such observations make it evident that it is impossible to say what is the safe minimum of any dietary factor, unless the biological values of all the other essential constituents of the diet are known. This represents an actual accomplishment of planning a diet which brings the animal into the "twilight" zone, where small shifts in the quality of the diet with respect to any factor may either distinctly stabilize the metabolic processes of the animal, or may lead to the development of a distinct pathologic state.

Their studies with the types of diets just described, lead them to the conclusion that it is unwise to approach very closely the physiological minimum with respect to any dietary factor. *Liberal consumption of all of the essential constituents of a normal diet, prompt digestion and absorption and prompt evacuation of the undigested residue from the intestine before ex-*

tensive absorption of products of bacterial decomposition of proteins can take place, are the optimum conditions for the maintenance of vigor and the characteristics of youth. Such a dietary régime can be attained only by supplementing the seed products, tubers, roots and meat, which must constitute the bulk of the diet of man, with the *protective foods*, milk and the leafy vegetables.

The results of the study of several representatives of each of the different classes of food-stuffs has led the author to the conclusion that, while it is not desirable to relegate to the background any of the fundamental knowledge of food-stuffs which can be obtained by chemical methods, and by respiration and digestion studies, the fundamental basis of nutrition can best be imparted to the public through the adoption of a biological classification of the natural food-stuffs on the basis of their function. Foods other than milk and eggs of both animal and vegetable origin may be arranged into groups according to whether they represent principally, functioning active protoplasm, or deposits of reserve food material, or in animal tissues, highly specialized contractile tissues. From their biological function their dietary properties can be fairly accurately predicted. This idea, together with the knowledge that milk, eggs and the leafy vegetables, the *protective foods*, are so constituted as to correct the dietary deficiencies of the seeds, tubers, roots and meat, should form the central idea in the teaching of the science of nutrition. It should be emphasized that the diet is a relatively complex thing, and that none of the essential constituents can be ignored in its planning, but that the observance of certain general rules of procedure will insure that any faults in the diet will be reduced to a minimum.

It is of special moment at this time to emphasize the importance of the dairy industry in its relation to the public health. Mankind may be roughly classified into two groups. Both of these have derived the greater part of their food supply from seeds, tubers, roots and meat, but have differed in respect to the character of the remainder of their diets. One group, represented by the Chinese, Japanese and the peoples of the Tropics generally, have employed the leaves of plants as almost their sole protective food. They likewise eat eggs and these serve to correct their diet. The other group includes the peoples of Europe and North America and a few others. These have likewise made use of the leaves of plants, but in lesser degree, and have, in addition, derived a very considerable part of their food supply from milk and its products.

Those peoples who have employed the leaf of the plant as their sole protective food are characterized by small stature, relatively short span of life, high infant mortality, and by contended adherence to the employment of the simple mechanical inventions of their forefathers. The peoples who have made liberal use of milk as a food, have, in contrast, attained greater size, greater longevity, and have been much more successful in the rearing of their young. They have been more aggressive than the non-milk using peoples, and have achieved much greater advancement in literature, science and art. They have developed in a higher degree educational and political systems which offer the greatest opportunity for the individual to develop his powers. Such development has a physiological basis, and there seems every reason to believe that it is fundamentally related to nutrition.

In the United States, we have in the past derived no less than 15 to 20 per cent of our total food supply from the products of the dairy. The investigations of recent years have thrown a new light on the importance of this increment of our diet. It has become evident that milk is the greatest factor of safety in our nutrition, and it is certain that we could not have accomplished what we have, had we dispensed with milk as a food.

The situation of the dairy industry is at the present time precarious. The cost of feeding-stuffs and of labor have enormously increased during the last few years, and consequently the cost of milk production. Advance in the cost of milk to the consumer has been made unavoidable. Every advance in the price has, however, met with great resistance by the public, and with each rise there has been a distinct drop in the amount purchased. The milk delivered in the city of Chicago has fallen off from about a million and a quarter quarts daily to about seven hundred thousand quarts, within a year. Similar reductions in sales have occurred almost everywhere in the Eastern half of the country, solely because of the rise in price. This has resulted in the discouragement of producers everywhere, and in a movement toward the reduction of the number of dairy cows.

There can be no doubt that there is great lack of knowledge by the people generally as to the importance of milk and other dairy products in the diet. There is no substitute for milk, and its use should be distinctly increased instead of diminished, regardless of cost. Every possible means should be employed to reduce the cost of distribution. The necessity for the liberal use of milk and its products both in the diets of children and adults should be emphasized in order to stem the ebbing tide of its production. It has been pointed out that the value of milk as a food cannot be estimated on the basis of its content of protein and energy. Even when measured by this standard it compares most favorably with other foods, but it has a value as a protective food, in improving the quality of the diet, which can be estimated only in terms of health and efficiency.

An examination of any large groups of people in the cities, will show that where there is a high mortality from tuberculosis, milk is not being used to any great extent, and in any large group where milk purchases are large this disease is not a menace.

It is well known that in institutions where tuberculosis is successfully treated milk forms the principal article of the diet of the inmates. This has resulted from clinical experience. There is no other effective treatment for this disease than that of providing fresh air, insisting upon rest and of heightening the body's powers of resistance through the liberal use of milk for the correction of faults which the diet will inevitably have when it consists too largely of seed products, tubers, roots and meats. The importance of diets of this character in the etiology of tuberculosis, has not hitherto been appreciated. In the light of facts presented in the previous chapters of this book, there can be no reasonable doubt that the importance of poor hygienic conditions and of poor ventilation have been greatly over-estimated, and that of poor diet not at all adequately appreciated as factors in promoting the spread of this disease. Milk is just as necessary in the diet of the adult as in that of the growing child. Any diet which will not support normal development in the young will not support optimum well-being in the adult. Milk is our greatest protective food, and its use must be increased. The price must be allowed to go up, so long as the cost of production makes it necessary, and up so far as is essential to make milk production a profitable business. Unless this is done, the effects will soon become apparent in a lowering of our standards of health and efficiency.

INTRODUCTION TO THE LEGENDS TO THE CHARTS

The data upon which the foregoing discussion of diet is based, consists of about three thousand feeding experiments. Most of these were carried out with domestic rats, but in order to demonstrate the general applicability of the results of tests made on one species to other species of animals, numerous feeding tests were made on farm pigs, cattle, chickens, guinea pigs and a few on pigeons. These all indicate that the chemical requirements of these different types of animals are essentially the same. The following charts present the growth curves of rats, fed a series of diets which illustrate the type of results from which the conclusions in this book are drawn. In each case the curve is the actual record of an individual which fairly represents the behavior of from four to six or more animals.

The broken curve marked N with the sex sign (σ = male; φ = female) represents the normal expectation of growth in each sex when fed a mixed diet containing several seeds and a liberal supply of milk. Vertically the curves designate body weight; horizontally from left to right the charts record duration of experiment, each square representing four weeks. A break in a curve marked **Y**, indicates the birth of a litter of young.

Although experiments are described only for the wheat, rice and oat kernel among the seeds, similar records are available for all the more important seeds used as foods in America, and these warrant the statement that seeds as a class closely resemble each other in their dietary properties. A close resemblance likewise exists among the several leaves which have been studied, so that the edible leaves may be regarded as having in a general way the same dietary properties.

CHART 1.—Lot 417 shows the results of restricting young rats to a diet of purified protein, salts, carbohydrate and agar-agar, together with an extract of a natural food-stuff which furnishes the dietary factor, water-soluble B, the substance which prevents beri-beri. The diet was complete except for the absence of the fat-soluble A. As a rule there develops in animals so fed, a type of xerophthalmia, which is due to the lack of the fat-soluble A. When a fat or other natural food which is rich in cellular structures (as contrasted with reserve food materials), is added to a food mixture of this type, the resulting diet becomes capable of inducing growth.

Lot 418, Period 1, shows the curves of body weight of rats fed a diet similar to that described above for Lot 417, but differing in that it contained butter fat (fat-soluble A) but lacked the extract of natural foods, and, therefore, contained no water-soluble B. On this diet xerophthalmia does not develop, but the animals ultimately lose muscular control and manifest symptoms suggestive of beri-beri in man. Growth is not possible on this diet, but everything which is needed in the diet so far as chemical analysis could show, is present.

These results show the necessity of a *biological analysis* of food-stuffs. Growth at once took place when, in Period 2, the dietary essential water-soluble B, which is likewise soluble in alcohol, was added to the diet. This dietary factor is abundant in all natural

CHART 1.

LOT 417
Ration:
Casein 18.0
Salts 3.7
Agar-agar 2.0
Dextrin 76.3
The dextrin carried the hot water extract of 11 grams of wheat embryo.

LOT 418
Ration:
Period 1
Casein 18.0
Salts 3.7
Agar-agar 2.0
Dextrin 71.3
Butter fat 5.0
Period 2
Part of the dextrin carried the alcoholic extract of 10 grams of wheat embryo.

LOT 419
Ration:
Casein 18.0
Agar-agar 2.0
Salts 3.7
Butter fat 5.0
Dextrin 71.3
The dextrin carried the cold water extract (subsequently freed from protein by coagulation by heat) of 15.9 grams of wheat embryo.

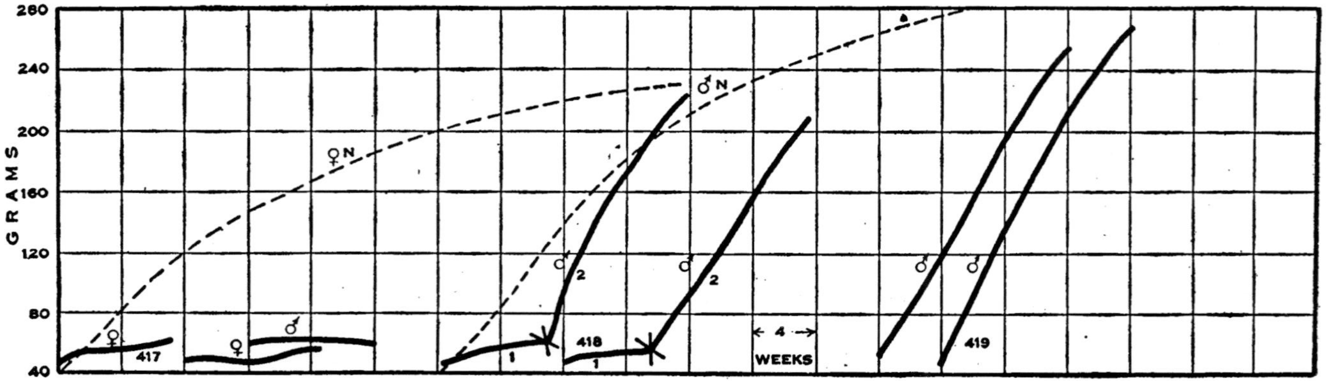

foods. In investigations of the nature of those here described, it is usually added as an alcoholic extract of a natural food.

Lot 419 shows the type of growth curves secured with diets containing both fat-soluble A and water-soluble B, in addition to the long recognized food substances, protein, carbohydrate, fat and a satisfactory supply of the inorganic elements essential for the nutrition of an animal. There is much reason to believe that each of the two unidentified dietary factors A and B contains but a single chemical complex which is physiologically indispensable, and not a group of such substances.

CHART 2.—This chart illustrates the nature of the dietary deficiencies of the cereal grains, as revealed by feeding a single variety of seed with the *addition* of certain purified food substances. Wheat is a typical representative of the group of seeds.

The wheat kernel when fed as the sole source of nutriment, or when supplemented with protein alone or with fat-soluble A alone (in butter fat), does not induce any growth in a young animal. Wheat supplemented with the three inorganic elements, calcium, sodium and chlorine, and with no other additions, induces slow growth for a time. In other words, the salt content is the first limiting factor in seeds from the dietary standpoint. These facts are not illustrated by growth curves.

Lot 223 illustrates the growth of young rats when fed wheat together with two purified food additions, viz., protein and a salt mixture of suitable composition. The dextrinized starch in this diet has no special significance. On this diet animals may grow to nearly the full adult size at the normal rate, and in some cases a small litter of young may be produced. The young as a rule will be allowed to die within a few days. On such a diet xerophthalmia will ultimately develop, and this forms the terminal event in the lives of the animals. This shows that the content of fat-soluble A in wheat is below the amount required to maintain an animal in a state of health over a long period. This fact is further illustrated by the record of rat 223-B, whose diet was like that of 223, except that the former contained 5 per cent of butter fat. Butter fat is the best known source of fat-soluble A.

Lot 380, Period 1, shows how slowly growth proceeds when the diet consists of wheat, supplemented with two purified food additions, protein and fat-soluble A (as butter fat). The deficiency of

CHART 2.

LOT 223
Ration:
Wheat   64.0
Casein   13.4
Salts   4.8
Dextrin   17.8

LOT 380
Ration, Period 1
Wheat   82.0
Casein   13.0
Butter fat   5.0
Period 2
4.8 per cent of salts
was added to the ration.

LOT 223–B
Ration:
Wheat   64.0
Casein   13.4
Dextrin   12.8
Salts   4.8
Butter fat   5.0

LOT 319
Ration:
Wheat   84.5
Salts   10.5
Butter fat   5.0

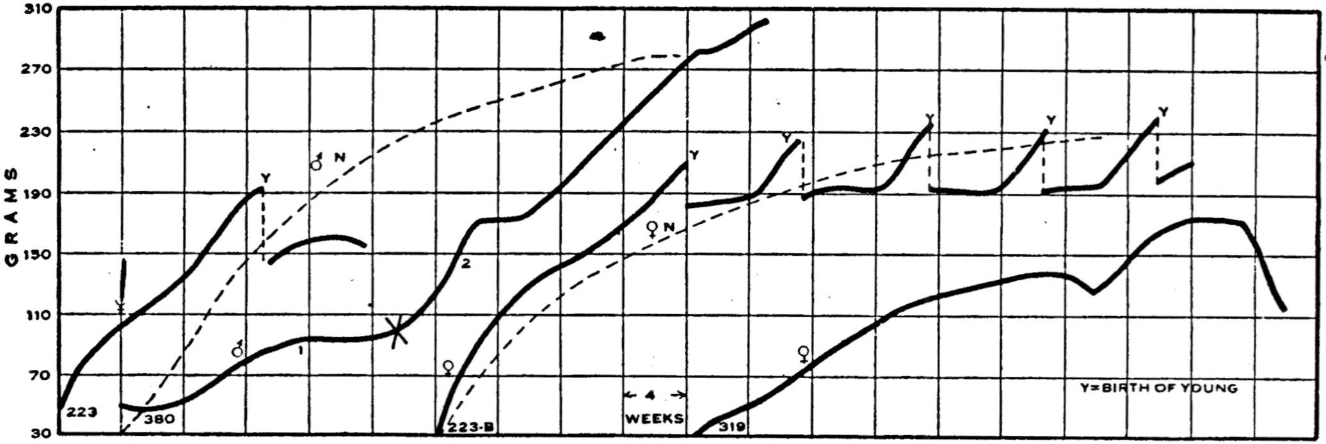

Y = BIRTH OF YOUNG

WEEKS

GRAMS

310   270   230   190   150   110   70   30

223   380   223-B   319

the wheat kernel in certain inorganic elements is illustrated by the great acceleration of growth in Period 2, when a suitably constituted salt mixture was added to the diet of Period 1.

Lot 319 shows the slow growth of a rat when fed wheat supplemented only with the requisite inorganic salts and fat-soluble A. The proteins of the wheat kernel are not of very good quality, and must be enhanced by further protein additions before growth can be normal.

Lot 223-B illustrates the fact that the optimum rate of growth is secured with wheat supplemented with three purified food additions, viz., salts, fat-soluble A and protein. When wheat is improved with respect to these three dietary factors, it becomes a complete food, and supports the production of the normal number of young, and the young are successfully reared. What is true of wheat is likewise true in a general way of the other seeds. Seeds are similar in their dietary properties. In other words, the mineral content of any seed must be improved by suitable salt additions, its protein content must be enhanced by the addition of other proteins which yield in greater abundance those amino-acids which it yields in small amounts, and in most cases additional fat-soluble A must be added in order to prevent the ultimate development of a pathological condition of the eyes. A liberal supply of milk will correct all the deficiencies of a seed diet.

CHART 3.—In the process of polishing, both the germ and the bran layer of the rice kernel are rubbed off, thus removing the cellular structures and leaving only the endosperm. This consists almost entirely of proteins, starch, a small amount of fats, and of mineral elements in the form of salts. Its proteins are of relatively low value for inducing growth. Polished rice is, therefore, practically comparable, from the dietary standpoint, to the diet of purified foodstuffs described in Chart 1.

Lot 317 shows the behavior of young rats which were fed polished rice supplemented with two dietary factors, viz., a suitable salt mixture and fat-soluble A. This does not support growth, since the diet is still deficient in two respects. It lacks the second dietary essential, water-soluble B, and its proteins are of too poor quality for the support of growth in the amount supplied by 90 per cent of rice. Such a diet as that of Lot 317 will permit the development of a condition in rats similar to beri-beri in man.

CHART 3.

Lot 317
Ration:
Polished rice 91.0
Salts 4.0
Butter fat 5.0

Lot 324
Ration:
Polished rice 64.0
Casein 13.4
Dextrin 10.8
Salts 4.8
Agar-agar 2.0
Butter fat 5.0

Lot 383
Ration:
Unpolished rice 88.0
Casein 5.0
Salts 2.0
Butter fat 5.0

Lot 401
Ration:
Polished rice 64.0
Casein 13.4
Salts 2.4
Dextrin 13.2
Agar-agar 2.0
Butter fat 5.0
The dextrin carried the alcoholic extract of 15.9 grams of wheat embryo.

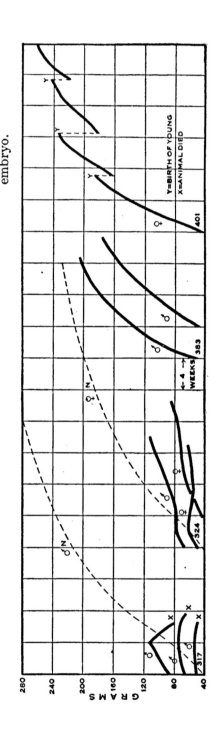

Lot 324 shows the effects on young rats of feeding them on a mixture consisting of polished rice supplemented with purified protein, a suitable salt mixture and fat-soluble A. The polished rice evidently contains some cellular elements and, therefore, some of the water-soluble B, for the animals were able to grow very slowly in some cases, and to remain alive during several months. Lot 401 illustrates the remarkable effects of adding to this diet an alcoholic extract of wheat germ. This extract furnished a liberal amount of water-soluble B (likewise soluble in alcohol) and renders the diet complete. The alcohol was employed to dissolve this dietary essential from the germ, and was evaporated completely before the ration was fed.

Lot 383 shows the dietary properties of unpolished as contrasted with polished rice. The former which contains the cellular structures of the germ and the bran layer, is rendered complete as a food by the addition of protein, fat-soluble A and salts. Young rats do not grow at all when fed solely upon unpolished rice, without these additions. Unpolished rice closely resembles wheat, corn, rye, barley and other seeds in its dietary properties.

Lot 401 shows the behavior of young animals when fed polished rice supplemented in four respects, viz., protein, a suitable salt mixture, fat-soluble A and water-soluble B. On this diet, young rats grew to the normal adult size, reproduced repeatedly and were able to rear a few of their young. The omission of any one of these additions would lead to almost complete failure of young animals to develop on this diet.

These examples make clear the method of procedure in making a biological analysis of a food-stuff. The latter consists of a suitably planned series of feeding experiments in which single and multiple purified food additions are made to a single natural food-stuff, and observations are made as to the ability of young animals to grow and perform the functions of adult life on the resulting food mixtures. In this way information can be secured which chemical methods are unable to reveal.

CHART 4.—These records illustrate the biological analysis of the dietary properties of the oat kernel (rolled oats). Lots 623 and 654 show the failure of young rats to grow on rolled oats supplemented with either a suitable inorganic mixture, or with purified protein as the only addition. Correction of these factors is necessary, but

CHART 4.

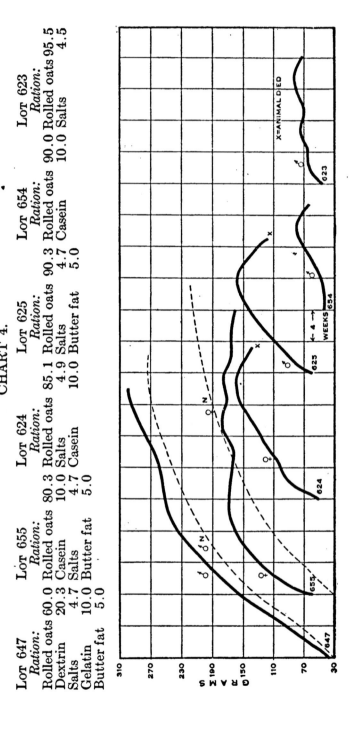

Lot 647
Ration:
Rolled oats 60.0
Dextrin 20.3
Salts 4.7
Gelatin 10.0
Butter fat 5.0

Lot 655
Ration:
Rolled oats 80.3
Salts 10.0
Casein 4.7
Butter fat 5.0

Lot 624
Ration:
Rolled oats 85.1
Salts 4.9
Butter fat 10.0

Lot 625
Ration:
Rolled oats 90.3
Casein 4.7
Butter fat 5.0

Lot 654
Ration:
Rolled oats 90.0
Casein 10.0

Lot 623
Ration:
Rolled oats 95.5
Salts 4.5

there are still other faults in the oat kernel which must be corrected before it becomes a complete food.   This is illustrated by the remaining records in this chart.

Lot 625 shows that when the oat kernel is supplemented with both a suitable salt mixture and fat-soluble A, it can support growth at a good rate for three months, but does not permit the animal to reach full adult size, and leads to early failure.   The protein of the oat kernel has a slightly higher value for growth than has that of either wheat or corn, but the amount furnished by 90 per cent of rolled oats is below the optimum for the support of growth in a rapidly growing species.   A diet rich in rolled oats produces very hard, pasty feces, which are difficult of elimination.   This appears to be a factor of importance in preventing the normal development of the experimental animals in this series.

Lot 624 further illustrates the inadequacy of rolled oats supplemented with both a suitable salt mixture and protein (casein). This food mixture lacks a sufficient amount of fat-soluble A, and unless there is an addition of this substance, the animals always develop the eye trouble (xerophthalmia) described on page 87.

Lot 655, shows the growth curve of an animal fed rolled oats supplemented with protein, an appropriate mineral salt mixture and fat-soluble A.   In this case the protein employed was casein of milk. This ration is dietetically complete, so far as its chemical composition is involved, but it did not support normal development to the full adult size.   It is not possible to state just how far the stunting was due to the pasty character of the feces formed from this diet, and how far the results should be attributed to the failure of casein to supplement the amino-acid deficiencies of the oat proteins.   Much better nutrition is secured with this diet when the casein is replaced by another protein, gelatin, as is shown by the records of Lot 647.

Lot 647 illustrates the completeness of a diet derived from rolled oats supplemented with an appropriate salt mixture, fat-soluble A and the protein, gelatin.   When Charts 2, 3 and 4 are compared, they show the striking similarity from the dietary standpoint of the three seeds, wheat, rice (unpolished) and oat kernels.

It is not to be concluded from these experiments which show the faulty character of these seeds as foods, that they are undesirable constituents of the diet.   Neither is it necessary or practicable to supplement in practice the seeds which we eat with additions of

CHART 5.

Lot 722
Ration:
Period 1
Flaxseed oil
  meal 10.0
Maize 90.0
Period 2
3.7 per cent of salts
replaced part of the
maize.

Lot 713
Ration:
Period 1
Millet seed 20.0
Rolled oats 20.0
Maize 20.0
Wheat 20.0
Hempseed 20.0
Period 2
3.7 per cent of
salts was added to
the mixture.

Lot 959
Ration:
Period 1
Wheat 31.0
Rolled oats 31.0
Maize 31.0
Dextrin 2.0
Butter fat 5.0
Period 2
1.0 per cent of
NaCl and 0.9 per-
cent of CaCO₃ re-
placed the dextrin.

Lot 1012
Ration:
Period 1
Wheat 28.0
Rolled oats 28.0
Maize 28.0
Casein 10.0
Dextrin 2.0
Butter fat 4.0
Period 2
1.0 per cent of
NaCl and 0.9 per
cent of CaCO₃ re-
placed the dextrin.

Lot 714-B
Ration:
Period 1
Maize 33.3
Rolled oats 33.3
Wheat 33.3
Period 2
5.0 per cent of
butter fat was
added to the ration.

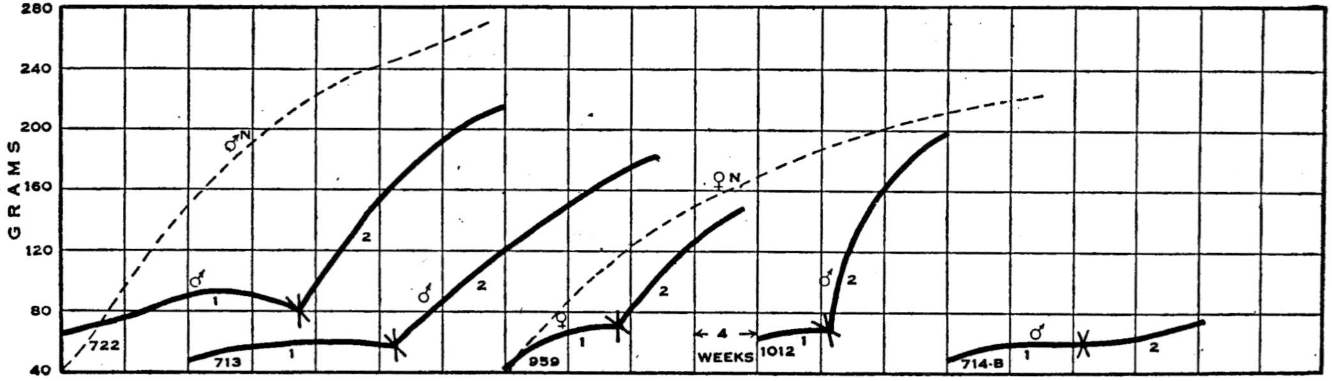

protein, salts, etc., in the manner employed in the biological analysis of these which we have described. There are two classes of *protective foods*, milk and the leafy vegetables, which when taken along with the seeds and their products, make good their deficiencies, and render the diet complete. *These correct the inorganic deficiencies (calcium, sodium and chlorine), insure a sufficient amount of fat-soluble A, and enhance the value of the proteins of the seed.*

CHART 5.—Each of the more important seeds which are employed in human and animal nutrition, have been studied by the methods employed for wheat, rice and the oat kernel, and the results show that the seeds all resemble each other in a general way in their dietary properties. They all require the same kinds of supplementary additions to make them complete foods. It would be expected, therefore, that mixtures of any seeds should not form complete diets. The following experiments demonstrate that this is indeed the case.

Lot 722 shows the failure of animals to grow when confined to a mixture of corn and flaxseed oil meal. After nearly four months of stunting there was an immediate response with growth when the inorganic content of the diet was supplemented with a suitable salt mixture.

Mixtures of seeds will, in nearly all cases, furnish proteins in greater value than those of the individual seeds fed singly, since the amino-acids in which they are relatively deficient are not the same in different seeds. The seeds all contain some of the fat-soluble A, but not as much as is desirable in the diet. In seed mixtures there is only a relative shortage of this dietary essential. The deficiency of certain inorganic elements is, therefore, the first limiting factor in mixtures of seeds as food-stuffs. In many of the growth curves exhibited in the charts, complex salt mixtures were added, since at the time the experiments were carried out, our knowledge concerning the inorganic factor was still very incomplete. It is now known that but three elements need be added to seed mixtures, viz., calcium, sodium and chlorine.

Lot 713 shows the failure of five seeds to support growth. In Period 2, the correction of the inorganic deficiencies of the diet was followed by a prompt response with growth. The poor quality of the proteins and relative shortage of fat-soluble A, will in time lower the vitality of animals fed such a seed mixture, when only the inorganic factor is corrected.

CHART 6.

LOT 685
Ration:
Rolled oats 60.0
Alfalfa   40.0

LOT 687
Ration:
Wheat   60.0
Alfalfa 40.0

LOT 686
Ration:
Maize   60.0
Alfalfa 40.0

LOT 478
Ration:
Rice   60.0
Alfalfa 40.0

LOT 688
Ration:
Peas (heated) 60.0
Alfalfa   40.0

LOT 717
Ration:
Cottonseed
flour   60.0
Alfalfa 40.0

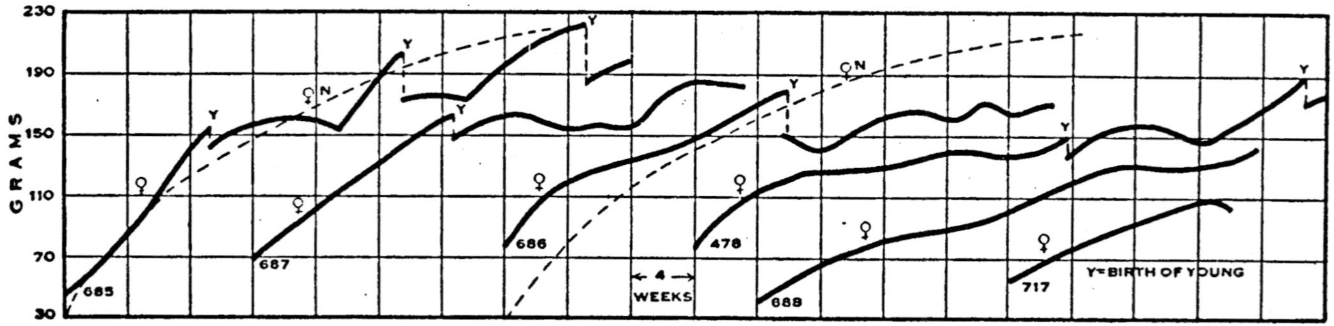

Lot 959 shows that the addition of fat-soluble A (as butter fat) to a mixture of three seeds, wheat, corn and oats, does not produce a food which can support growth except at a very slow rate. In Period 2, the correction of the inorganic deficiencies of the diet was followed by a prompt response with growth.

Lot 1012, in Period 1, received three seeds supplemented with both protein (casein) and fat-soluble A, but could not grow on this diet. In Period 2, the addition of the necessary salts produced an immediate response with growth.

Lot 714-B, which were fed three seeds, suffered complete suspension of growth. There was no response in Period 2, to the addition of fat-soluble A in butter fat. Although both protein and fat-soluble A are desirable additions to any seed diet, and are necessary before the optimum nutrition can be attained, the inorganic deficiencies must be corrected before any noticeable benefit can be derived from the correction of the other factors. (Compare 959–714-B.)

CHART 6.—In marked contrast to the failure of young animals to grow on a diet restricted to seeds, one can secure very satisfactory rations from mixtures of leaf and seed. The leaf is a cell rich structure; the seed, a cell poor storage organ. With this difference in function go corresponding differences in dietary properties. (See pages 43–44.)

These curves illustrate the relative values for the support of growth and reproduction of diets derived from alfalfa leaf flour 40 per cent, and a seed 60 per cent. It will be seen that these corresponding leaf and seed mixtures are not of equal value. In a general way the leaves all resemble each other in their dietary properties, and form a distinct group of food-stuffs as do the seeds.

Lot 685 shows the possibility of securing a normal growth curve and repeated reproduction with a rat restricted to a mixture of alfalfa leaf flour 40 per cent and rolled oats 60 per cent. Of the six litters (33 young) borne by mothers which had grown up on this diet, 16 young or 50 per cent were successfully reared to weaning time. Despite the fact that an animal can grow at a rate which we may regard as normal on this food mixture, it is not of a highly satisfactory character. Rolled oats and alfalfa leaf make a better diet than the alfalfa leaf with any other seed which we have studied. It is interesting that these proportions between alfalfa leaf and rolled oats give better results in the nutrition of the rat than any others.

CHART 7.

Lot 273
Ration:
Maize   50.0
Alfalfa leaf 30.0
Peas (heated) 20.0

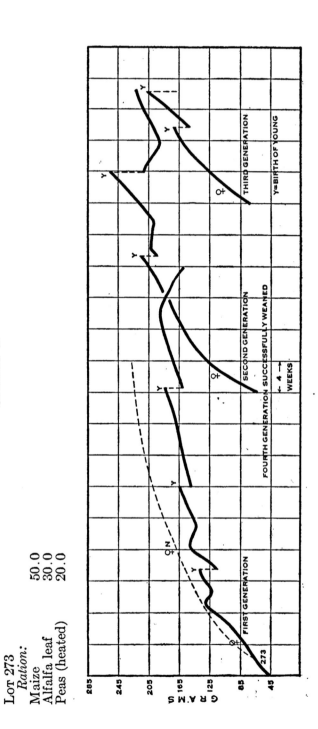

Lots 687 and 686, show that there is little difference in the values of mixtures of the alfalfa leaf with the wheat kernel as compared with the corn kernel. Both, in the proportions here employed, fail to induce growth at the "normal" rate, and the number of young produced was approximately one-fifth that which a female rat will produce when her diet is of excellent quality. A well-nourished female rat may be expected to produce five litters of young.

Lot 478 shows that even with a simple mixture of alfalfa leaf flour 40 per cent and polished rice 60 per cent, rats were able to grow to about 83 per cent of the normal adult size and to produce young. The rat whose curve is shown had two litters. All young from mothers which had grown up on this diet were allowed to die during the first few days after birth.

Lots 688 and 717, show that combinations of peas or of cottonseed with the alfalfa leaf flour form food mixtures which can support growth at a slow rate, but are inferior to certain other combinations of leaf and seed.

There are very great possibilities for improving our practices in the utilization of feeding-stuffs in animal production. We need exact knowledge regarding the best combinations and proportions in which to feed our natural products.

CHART 7.—It is easily possible to prepare diets which are derived solely from vegetable sources, which will induce growth from weaning time to full adult size and support the production of young. Success in this direction involves the employment of suitable combinations of leaves, together with foods of plant origin whose functions are. those of storage organs, viz.: seeds, tubers, and roots. The records here presented show the most successful results which we have obtained with mixtures of leaf and seeds.

Lot 273 shows the results of restricting young rats from weaning time to a diet derived entirely from the alfalfa leaf flour, corn and peas. The peas were cooked at 15 pounds pressure for one hour in an autoclave. The other constituents of the diet were fed raw.

The female rat marked, First Generation, never grew to the full adult size, but others in the same cage with her did. The curve of this particular rat is presented because she became the great grand-mother of a litter whose ascendants for four generations ate, beyond the weaning age, nothing but this monotonous mixture of vegetable foods.

CHART 8.

Lot 652
Ration:
Wheat 70.0
Dextrin 10.0
Salts 5.0
Gelatin 10.0
Butter fat 5.0

Lot 493
Ration:
Wheat 70.0
Dextrin 20.0
Salts 5.0
Butter fat 5.0

Lot 647
Ration:
Rolled Oats 60.0
Dextrin 20.3
Salts 4.7
Gelatin 10.0
Butter fat 5.0

Lot 646
Ration:
Rolled Oats 60.0
Dextrin 30.3
Salts 4.7
Butter fat 5.0

Lot 756
Ration:
Period 1
Peas 45.0
Gelatin 9.0
Salts 1.9
Agar-agar 1.0
Dextrin 38.1
Butter fat 5.0
Period 2
9 per cent of casein
replaced gelatin.

Lot 785
Ration:
Same as 756 with
beans in place of
peas.

Lot 651
Ration:
Maize 71.3
Dextrin 18.0
Salts 3.7
Agar-agar 2.0
Butter fat 5.0

Lot 649
Ration:
Maize 71.3
Dextrin 8.0
Salts 3.7
Gelatin 10.0
Butter fat 5.0
Agar-agar 2.0

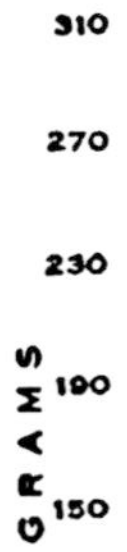

310

270

230

190

150

GRAMS

This ration did not induce optimum nutrition. The number of young produced was approximately half what well-fed rats normally produce, and the mortality of the young was high. Although the breeding records were poor and the litters small, most of these young were reared. Notwithstanding this, the vigor of the fourth generation appeared to be as great as that of the first.

The above mixture gives better results in the nutrition of the rat than any other proportions in which these three food-stuffs can be combined. If the amount of alfalfa leaf is raised to 40 per cent or reduced to 20 per cent, and the content of corn is reduced or increased respectively, few young will be reared. The importance of knowing the exact proportions in which to combine our natural food-stuffs in order to secure the optimum results in nutrition, especially in animal production, will be evident from these results.

CHART 8.—This chart affords an illustration of the great differences in the degree in which a supplementary addition of protein may enhance the value of the proteins of a natural food-stuff. The curves should be considered in pairs.

Lot 493 shows the results of feeding a diet deriving its protein content entirely from the wheat kernel. The diet contained but 7 per cent of protein, an amount too small because of the relatively poor quality of the wheat proteins, to support growth at the optimum rate. The group of rats which were fed this diet grew at about half the normal rate.

Lot 652 received the same diet, with 10 per cent of the carbohydrate replaced by the protein gelatin. The latter is one of the "incomplete" proteins, since it lacks three of the amino-acids which are essential for the nutrition of an animal. A diet which contains gelatin as its sole protein, no matter how much gelatin it may contain, cannot induce any growth whatever in a young animal. Lot 652, however, grew at the optimum rate. This result shows that the added gelatin made good a limited supply of certain amino-acids in the wheat proteins of the diet. This formed the limiting factor in determining the slow rate of growth in Lot 493. Gelatin is shown by this experiment to supplement well the proteins of the wheat kernel.

Lots 756 and 785, show the stunting of young rats fed diets which derived their protein entirely from a mixture of peas and gelatin, and a mixture of navy beans and gelatin respectively. Both diets contained about 18 per cent of protein. When of good quality this

CHART 9.

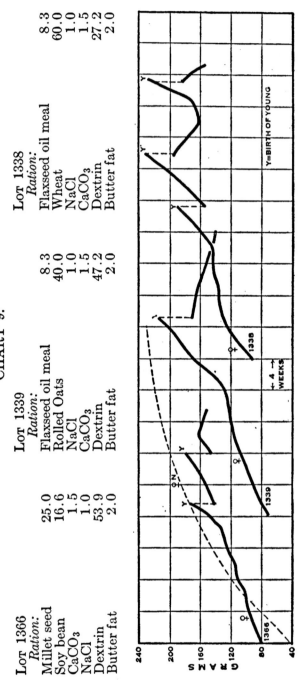

LOT 1366		LOT 1339		LOT 1338	
Ration:		*Ration:*		*Ration:*	
Millet seed	25.0	Flaxseed oil meal	8.3	Flaxseed oil meal	8.3
Soy bean	16.6	Rolled Oats	40.0	Wheat	60.0
CaCO₃	1.5	NaCl	1.0	NaCl	1.0
NaCl	1.0	CaCO₃	1.5	CaCO₃	1.5
Dextrin	53.9	Dextrin	47.2	Dextrin	27.2
Butter fat	2.0	Butter fat	2.0	Butter fat	2.0

amount suffices for the support of normal growth. Combinations of pea proteins with gelatin, and of bean proteins with gelatin, yield amino-acid mixtures which are deficient in some way.

In Period 2 in both cases, the diets differed from those of Period 1, only in that the gelatin was replaced by an equal amount of casein from milk. This change led to great improvement in the quality of the protein in the diets, and growth at once proceeded at a good rate. Gelatin does not greatly enhance the value of the proteins of either the pea or the bean, whereas casein does.

Lots 646 and 647 show the effect on growth, of feeding a diet containing but 9 per cent of protein derived solely from rolled oats (Lot 646), and the same diet with 10 per cent of carbohydrate replaced by gelatin. In the former case, growth was early suspended, but in the latter, growth proceeded at the optimum rate to full maturity. This result shows that gelatin supplements the proteins of the oat kernel in a very satisfactory manner. (See discussion under Lots 493 and 652.)

Lots 649 and 651, show the growth curves of rats fed, in the former case a diet which derived its protein content of about 7 per cent entirely from the corn kernel, and in the latter case the same diet with 10 per cent of its carbohydrate replaced by gelatin. In marked contrast to the effects of feeding gelatin together with wheat or oat proteins, there is no improvement in the quality of corn proteins through combining these with gelatin. Gelatin does not supplement the peculiar amino-acid deficiencies of the corn kernel.

CHART 9.—The records in this chart give an idea of the values of the proteins derived from mixtures of two seeds. Each of the diets described contained 9 per cent of protein. It has been established that this content of protein in a ration, when it is derived from either the wheat, corn or rice kernel alone, does not support growth at a rate much faster than half the normal rate. We, therefore, fed a series of diets in which the protein content was adjusted at this level, and derived from combinations of two seeds, in order to find the most fortunate combinations of seeds as sources of proteins for growth. Normal growth is secured on diets of this character, only in those cases where the proteins of one seed enhance those of the other seed present in the diet. We have not been able to find any two seeds whose proteins, when fed together even approximate the value of the proteins of milk.

CHART 10.

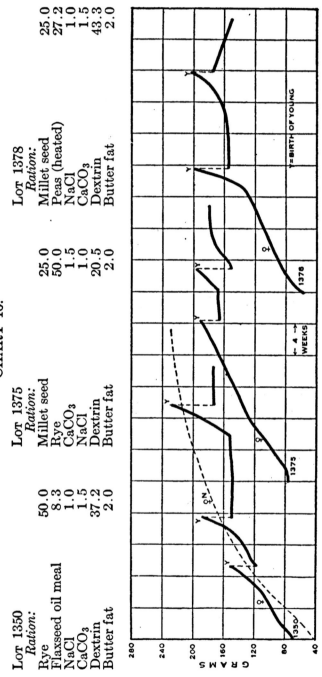

LOT 1350
Ration:
Rye 50.0
Flaxseed oil meal 8.3
NaCl 1.0
CaCO₃ 1.5
Dextrin 37.2
Butter fat 2.0

LOT 1375
Ration:
Millet seed 25.0
Rye 50.0
CaCO₃ 1.5
NaCl 1.0
Dextrin 20.5
Butter fat 2.0

LOT 1378
Ration:
Millet seed 25.0
Peas (heated) 27.2
NaCl 1.0
CaCO₃ 1.5
Dextrin 43.3
Butter fat 2.0

Lot 1366, derived 3 per cent of protein from millet seed and 6 per cent from the soy bean. The deficiencies of the diet, aside from the character of the proteins, were all made good by suitable additions of salts and butter fat. On this diet the growth was slow, and the animals remained undersized. On this diet three females have produced four litters (23) young of which but three individuals were weaned, the others being allowed to die in infancy. This protein mixture is of relatively low biological value.

Lot 1339 derived 6 per cent of protein from rolled oats and 3 per cent from flaxseed oil meal. Two females grew up on this diet. One remained sterile, and the other produced but one litter of young (7). These were finally weaned after a long period of infancy in which their growth was very slow. They were very small and runty when weaned. A protein mixture derived from these two seeds is of relatively poor quality.

Lot 1338 derived 6 per cent of protein from the wheat kernel and 3 per cent from flaxseed oil meal. Growth was below the normal rate, and two females have produced but three litters (18) young. But five of these were successfully weaned. Proteins derived from these two seeds are of relatively low biological value. They sufficed for the support of a fair rate of growth, but not for the additional strain of reproduction. This mixture must have both protein and fat-soluble A additions in order to produce the optimum results in nutrition.

CHART 10.—Like the preceding chart, this shows the relative biological values of the protein mixtures derived from mixtures of two seeds. The diet was made adequate in every respect, except the protein, which was in all cases adjusted so as to form 9 per cent of the food mixture. The reason for this has been made clear in the discussion of Chart 9.

Lot 1350 derived 6 per cent of protein from rye, and 3 per cent from flaxseed oil meal. Growth fell slightly below the normal expectation. One female and her daughter have produced five litters (30) young, of which but five individuals have been reared. This diet is not quite satisfactory as is shown by the reproduction records, and because of the poor quality of its proteins, and shortage of fat-soluble A.

Lot 1375 secured 6 per cent of protein from rye and 3 per cent from millet seed. One female which grew up on this diet has had

CHART 11.

The basal food-mixture consisted of the following foodstuffs:

Casein 18.0
Salts 3.7
Agar-agar
Dextrin 2.0
Natural food

The individual groups received natural food additions as follows:

Lot 723	Lot 633	Lot 631
Flaxseed 20 per cent	Alfalfa leaf 20 per cent	*Period 1*
		Alfalfa leaf 5 per cent
Lot 716	Lot 632	*Period 2*
Millet seed 25 per cent	Alfalfa leaf 10 per cent	Alfalfa leaf 30 per cent

Lot 710
Hemp seed 15 per cent

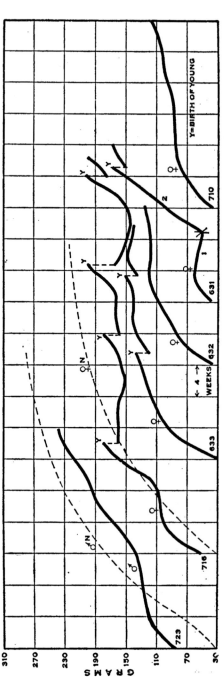

two litters of young, all of which were allowed to die in infancy. Another female remained sterile. It is evident that this combination of proteins does not form a fortunate mixture.

Lot 1378 derived 6 per cent of protein from peas and 3 per cent from millet seed. Growth on this diet was slower than the normal expectation, and reproduction was below normal. Two females produced four litters (17) of young, of which but nine individuals were finally weaned at an advanced age. These were very small for their age. Combinations of pea and millet seed proteins do not appear to have a very high biological value.

These histories selected from a long series of similar experiments in our records make it clear that it is not easy to find mixtures of two seeds whose proteins are of such a character as to supplement each other's deficiencies, in the yields of certain amino-acids, and produce mixtures of high biological value for growth and the promotion of physiological well-being. In order to demonstrate the effects of a limited protein content, or of proteins of poor quality in the diet, experiments must be continued over a relatively long period of time. Observations of man or animals on such diets may lead to faulty deductions when the experiments are of short duration.

Chart 11.—This chart illustrates in a general way the content of the two unidentified dietary essentials, fat-soluble A and water-soluble B, in certain natural foods. The diet in all cases consisted principally of purified food substances, and was adequate for the support of growth, except that its content of fat-soluble A and water-soluble B was derived from the small addition of natural food. As will appear from the records in Chart 12, these additions of natural food-stuffs, probably furnished a sufficient amount of water-soluble B to support normal growth, so it may fairly be said that these records afford more nearly an estimation of the content of fat-soluble A in each of the natural foods employed.

Lot 723 shows that 20 per cent of flaxseed does not supply enough of the fat-soluble A to support normal growth in a young rat.

Lot 716, shows that 25 per cent of millet seed supplied enough of both the unidentified dietary essentials for the support of nearly normal growth, and induced sufficiently good nutrition to make possible the production of nearly the normal number of young. The female rat usually produces five litters of young before she reaches the age of fourteen months, which age marks the end of her

CHART 12.

The basal food-mixture consisted of the following foodstuffs:

Casein	18.0
Salts	3.7
Butter fat	5.0
Dextrin	
Seed	
Agar-agar	2.0

The individual groups received natural food additions as follows:

Lot 676   Lot 475   Lot 645   Lot 695
Wheat 35 per cent Wheat 25 per cent Wheat 15 per cent Peas 25 per cent

Lot 696
Navy beans 25 per cent

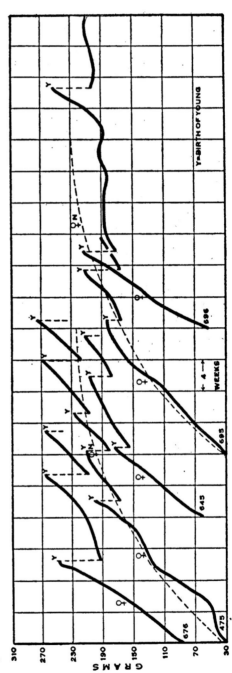

period of fertility. The rat whose curve is shown, had four litters during the first thirteen months of her life. The first two litters died early, but the third and fourth, which were born after butter fat (more fat-soluble A) was added to the mother's diet, were successfully brought to weaning age.

Lot 633, whose diet derived both the unidentified dietary essentials from its content of 20 per cent of alfalfa leaf, remained distinctly undersized, and produced but two litters of young, all of which died in early infancy.

Lot 632, which received but 10 per cent of alfalfa as its sole source of fat-soluble A and water-soluble B, grew slowly, and never reached a body weight greater than half the normal adult size, and produced no young.

Lot 631 was unable to grow at all when restricted to 5 per cent of alfalfa leaf as its sole source of both the unidentified dietary essentials, but responded at once with growth when the content of leaf was raised to 30 per cent.

Lot 710 failed to grow well when restricted to a diet which derived its fat-soluble A and water-soluble B from 15 per cent of hemp seed. The oil seeds, judging from the limited data available, seem to contain more of the fat-soluble A than do the cereal grains, but less than millet seed. The latter is richer in this substance than any other seed yet studied.

CHART 12.—These records were obtained with diets which derived their content of water-soluble B entirely from the amount of natural food-stuff which each contained. The basal diet consisted of purified protein, carbohydrate, a suitable mineral salt mixture, and butter fat to furnish the fat-soluble A. The curves give an approximate idea of the minimum amount of each of several natural food-stuffs which are necessary to furnish sufficient water-soluble B to enable a young rat to grow and reproduce.

Lots 645, 475 and 676 demonstrate the relative richness of the wheat kernel in water-soluble B. Even 15 per cent furnishes enough to enable a young rat to grow to approximately the full adult size, and to produce several litters of young. None can be successfully weaned on this diet. Even with 25 per cent of wheat in the diet, we have not seen a litter of young brought to the weaning age when the mother was restricted to this type of diet. When the wheat is increased to 35 per cent of the food mixture some young can be

CHART 13.

Lot 1414		
Ration:		
Potato		25.0
Peas		69.5
NaCl		1.0
CaCO$_3$		1.5
Butter fat		3.0

Lot 1423		
Ration:		
Period 1		
Potato		25.0
Peas		65.0
Casein		10.0
Period 2		

3 per cent of butter fat replaced an equivalent amount of peas.

Period 3

NaCl 1.0 and CaCO$_3$ 1.5 were added to the ration.

Lot 1450		
Ration:		
Period 1		
Potato		25.0
Peas		72.0
Butter fat		3.0
Period 2		

NaCl 1.0 and CaCO$_3$ 1.5 replaced part of the peas.

Lot 1405		
Ration:		
Potato		25.0
Peas		72.5
NaCl		1.0
CaCO$_3$		1.5

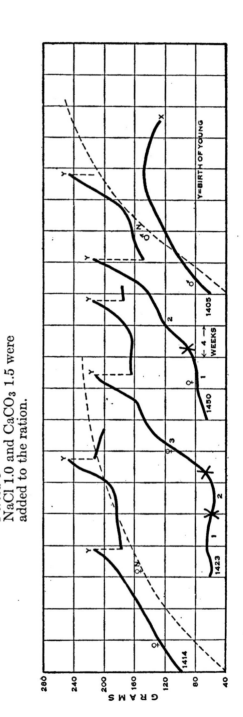

Y=BIRTH OF YOUNG

reared, but the mortality is still very high. With higher levels of wheat substituted for carbohydrate in this formula, the successful rearing of young becomes the rule.

Lot 695 shows that 25 per cent of cooked peas in the diet as the sole source of water-soluble B furnishes a sufficient amount of this substance to enable young rats to grow well and produce young. None were reared by any of the female rats in this lot. The peas were soaked in water and heated for an hour and a quarter in an autoclave at fifteen pounds pressure, dried and ground. This treatment is approximately the equivalent of the heat employed in the processing of canned fruits and vegetables. There seems to be little loss of water-soluble B as the result of such heating.

Lot 696 shows that 25 per cent of navy beans, which had been soaked and heated in a manner similar to that described for peas (Lot 695), supplied enough of water-soluble B to enable rats to grow to full adult size and reproduce. Eight young out of eighteen young (2 litters) were reared by mothers confined to this diet.

CHART 13.—It has been pointed out (page 46) that the tuber and the edible root are both storage organs, and, therefore, poor in cellular structures, and that their dietary properties are very closely similar to the seeds. The records of young rats which were fed mixtures of potato and peas, supplemented in various ways according to the biological method of food analysis, demonstrates the truth of this assertion.

Lot 1405 illustrates the slow growth and early death of a rat fed a mixture of peas and potato, supplemented with the mineral elements, calcium, sodium and chlorine. An inspection of the remaining curves in the chart reveals the fact that the diet is still deficient with respect to fat-soluble A, and in no other respect.

Lot 1450, Period 1, shows the failure of animals to grow when fed peas, potato and fat-soluble A. When in Period 2, pure sodium chloride (common salt) and calcium carbonate (chalk) were added, growth became possible at the normal rate. Two litters of young have been born and all were successfully weaned. This result indicates that the protein content derived from peas and potato is of satisfactory character, and this conclusion is supported by the records of Lot 1414, which has been successful in growth and reproduction when restricted to this protein mixture. To this mixture of peas and potato, both the inorganic content and the content of fat-

CHART 14.

Lot 1406	Lot 1415	Lot 1442	Lot 1397
Ration:	*Ration:*	*Ration:*	*Ration:*
	Period 1	*Period 1*	
Potato 25.0	Potato 25.0	Potato 25.0	Potato 25.0
Maize 69.5	Maize 65.0	Maize 72.0	Maize 72.5
NaCl 1.0	Casein 10.0	Butter fat 3.0	NaCl 1.0
CaCO₃ 1.5	*Period 2*	*Period 2*	CaCO₃ 1.5
Butter fat 3.0	3 per cent of butter	NaCl 1.0 and CaCO₃ 1.5	
	fat replaced part of	were added to the ration	
	maize.		
	Period 3		
	NaCl 1.0 and CaCO₃ 1.5		
	were added to the ration.		

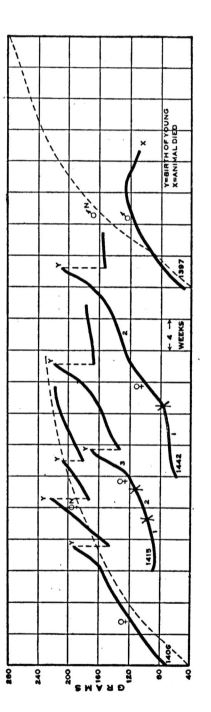

soluble A must be modified by suitable additions in order to make it dietetically complete.

Lot 1423, Period 1, shows failure of animals to grow on a diet of peas and potato supplemented with purified protein. In Period 2, fat-soluble A was added, but still growth could not take place. In Period 3, the addition of calcium, sodium and chlorine, rendered the diet complete. Two females have produced three litters (24) young, of which 16 have been successfully weaned, and the remaining ones are apparently normal, but under weaning age.

Lot 1414 shows that good growth and reproduction are possible on a diet derived from peas and potato, supplemented with the necessary salts and fat-soluble A, and gives an idea of the quality of the protein mixture derived from these sources. It is of interest to note that the proteins of the pea when taken in the amount furnished by this diet (about 18 per cent) and forming the sole proteins of the diet, do not support normal growth even when the diet is made complete with respect to all other factors. The proteins of the potato are of such a nature as to enhance the value of the proteins of the pea.

In preparing these food materials the potatoes were steamed, skinned, dried and ground. The peas were soaked, heated in an autoclave at fifteen pounds pressure for an hour and a half, dried and ground. The ingredients of the diet were ground so as to make it impossible for the rats to pick out and eat them separately.

CHART 14.—These records illustrate the dietary properties of a. mixture of the corn kernel and potato. Like the preceding chart they show that this mixture closely resembles a mixture of two seeds, and supports the view that the storage tissues of plants all resemble each other in their dietary properties.

Lot 1397 shows the failure of the animals to grow when fed a mixture of corn and potato supplemented with the only inorganic salts necessary to complete its mineral content. That no other elements are necessary is made clear by the records of the other animals in this chart.

Lot 1442, Period 1, shows that the addition of fat-soluble A, without salts, does not make growth possible on a mixture of potato and corn kernel. In Period 2, growth took place at once on the addition of sodium chloride and calcium carbonate.

Lot 1415, Periods 1 and 2, illustrate the fact that the addition of

CHART 15.

211—Normal
1978—Rolled Oats 60.0 + NaCl 1.0 + CaĊO₃ 1.5 + Dextrin 32.5 + Butter fat 5.0
899—Rolled Oats + Salts 4.7
983—Rolled Oats + Casein 18.0 + Butter fat 5.0
843—Rolled Oats + Butter fat 5.0
738—Rolled Oats 100.0

290·

250

210

170

130

90

50

10

300

260

220

GRAMS

protein (casein) alone, or of protein, and fat-soluble A, respectively, does not make the mixture of potato and corn kernel dietetically complete. In Period 3, when the necessary salts were added, growth took place at once. The rat whose curve is shown has successfully reared two litters of young (14) and her daughter, from the first litter, has weaned a litter of seven young. The daughter has been fed exclusively upon the diet of Period 3, since she was weaned. These results make it clear that this mixture of corn, casein, potato, butter fat and the two salts, forms a very satisfactory diet.

Lot 1406 shows the ability of young rats to grow and reproduce at the normal rate and rear part of their young when confined to a diet of corn and potato supplemented with fat-soluble A and two salts, calcium carbonate and sodium chloride. This record indicates that the proteins derived from these two sources are of fairly good biological value. The diet contains but 9 per cent of total crude protein (N x 6.25). If the protein were all derived from the corn kernel, this amount would not support such a good rate of growth, and no rearing of young.

From the data available in our records, it is apparent that the potato is a very valuable food, a conclusion which is in harmony with the favor in which it has come to be regarded as an article òf diet for man.

CHART 15.—This and the following chart describe the relation of the mother as a factor of safety in the nutrition of her young. In nearly all of these records the mother was fed during lactation, a diet which was faulty in some respect, and on whjch the young, after the weaning age, could not grow at all. The problem was to find to what extent the mother is able to take such faulty diets, and produce milk of a character which will support growth in her young. The results show that the mother is capable under such dietary limitations of providing for her offspring a better diet for growth than she herself receives.

The mothers were fed an excellent diet until they delivered their young. The litter was in all cases reduced to four, in order to make the results comparable, and in order not to place an excessive burden upon the mother. From the day the young were born the mother received the faulty experimental diet.

Rat 211 illustrates the rate of growth of a litter of four young when the diet of the mother is highly satisfactory. This diet contained a liberal amount of milk and of wheat, together with a salt mixture and butter fat.

Rat 738 was fed nothing but rolled oats. Young after being weaned cannot grow at all on this diet. During the first 20 days the young grew slowly, then became stunted, and died between the 40th and 50th days. There are three types of deficiency in rolled oats: the inorganic content is unsatisfactory, the content of fat-soluble A is very low, and the proteins are not of very high value for growth. Notwithstanding these deficiencies, the lactating mother was able to produce milk having considerable growth-promoting properties.

Rat 843 was fed rolled oats with one of its deficiencies corrected, viz: by the addition of fat-soluble A. The growth curve of her young shows that her milk was of distinctly better quality than that which she could have produced from oats alone. The young grew faster and growth continued over a longer interval. Since the young continued to grow to the 50th day, it is evident that the mother was still supplementing the diet of oats and butter fat, which they began to eat at about the 20th day of age, with a considerable amount of milk which corrected the inorganic content of the oat kernel, for without the addition of calcium, sodium and cholrine, rolled oats cannot support growth, even when its other deficiencies are corrected.

Rat 983 did no better with her young on a diet of oats to which both protein and fat-soluble A were added, than did rat 843, without the protein addition. The first limiting factor for the mother in milk production is the inorganic content, just as it is for growth in the young.

Rat 899 did remarkably well in inducing growth in her young when her diet consisted of rolled oats and a suitable addition of salts for the correction of the inorganic deficiencies of the oat kernel. The seed is not entirely free from fat-soluble A, and the mother seems to have a reserve supply of this substance in her tissues which she can, for a time, contribute to her milk.

Rat 1978, which was fed oats supplemented with salts and fat-soluble A, induced growth at a fairly good rate in her young. The 60 per cent of oats in her diet furnished but 9 per cent of protein, and this did not suffice, because of its relatively low value, for the production of a normal milk supply. The growth of these young after the time they became able to eat of the mother's food supply, was much more rapid than it would have been had they not been getting a supplementary milk supply from the mother during the period covered by the growth curve.

Chart 16 contains further records of the growth of young which were suckling mothers on diets derived from rolled oats, supplemented in various ways.

CHART 16.—Continuing the records described in Chart 15.

Rat 948 shows the failure of the young to develop beyond a limited degree on a diet of rolled oats supplemented with protein only. The behavior of these young is comparable to that of Lot 738, Chart 16. The two most serious deficiencies of the oat kernel for milk production as for growth in the young, are the inorganic factor and the shortage of fat-soluble A.

It was shown in Chart 8 that oat proteins combined with gelatin, form a highly satisfactory protein mixture. This is confirmed by the growth at half normal rate of the young of rat 949, whose diet consisted of rolled oats and gelatin. Young rats cannot grow at all on this mixture. The mother is able to take such a faulty diet, and furnish milk of such a character as will safeguard her young in a most remarkable degree. Her limitations are, however, easily apparent.

Rat 984 did slightly better in extending the lives of her young when she was fed rolled oats plus gelatin plus butter fat (fat-soluble A), than did rat 949, on the same food, minus the butter fat. It should be remembered that young rats cannot grow at all, if when, after being weaned, they are confined to this diet. The rôle of the mother as a factor of safety in the nutrition of her young is easily seen.

Rat 1020, which was fed oats, gelatin and salts, was limited only with respect to the relative shortage of fat-soluble A in her diet. Nevertheless, she was able to produce milk which could induce growth at a fairly good rate in her young.

Rat 1019, was fed a diet which differed from that of 1020 only in containing casein. This appears to have had a slightly beneficial effect.

Rat 980 was fed rolled oats plus 20 per cent of skim milk powder. This amount was not sufficient to correct the inorganic deficiencies of the diet, and failed to supply enough fat-soluble A to render the diet satisfactory for milk production. It seems probable that the sodium chloride content and fat-soluble A in the skim milk powder

CHART 16.

211—Normal
980—Rolled Oats 80.0 + Powdered skim milk 20.0
1019—Rolled Oats + Casein 18.0 + Salts 4.7
1020—Rolled Oats + Gelatin 10.0 + Salts 4.7
984—Rolled Oats + Gelatin 10 0 + Butter fat 5.0
949—Rolled Oats + Gelatin 10.0
948—Rolled Oats + Casein 18.0

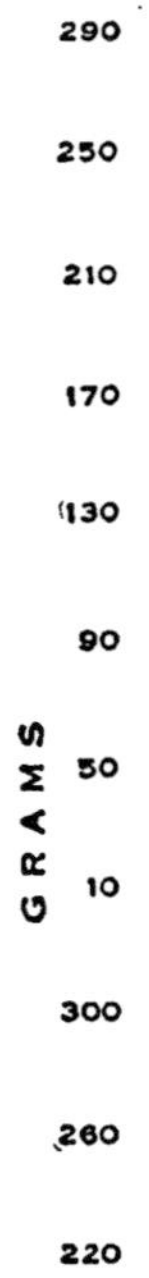

GRAMS

290 250 210 170 130 90 50 10 300 260 220

were the limiting factors in preventing the production of normal milk in this case.

In answer to the question as to whether the failure of the young to grow on the milk they received in these experiments, was not the result of insufficiency in quantity rather than quality of milk, we have the observations on cows, which were fed insufficient food during lactation, and in other experiments, in which cows were starved for common salt for periods of eight to fifteen months, and actually died or came near death from salt starvation. Under such conditions the milk flow was kept up over a long period in a most surprising manner.

We have further evidence that the young rats in the experiments described, continued in some instances to grow long after they became able to eat of their mother's food, when the latter was of such a character as to permit of no growth whatever, had it not been supplemented with a considerable amount of milk from the mother. When it is considered that in some of these cases the young weighed more than half as much as the mother, it must be admitted that the milk production, even in these greatly prolonged periods of lactation, while the mothers were taking faulty diets, must have been very considerable.

The relation between the character of the diet of the nursing mother and the character of the milk she produces has been discussed in Chapter 6.

BIBLIOGRAPHY

Chapter I

1. Fischer: Chemistry of the Proteins, Mann.
2. Osborne, T. B.: The Vegetable Proteins. Monographs on Biochemistry, Longmans, Green and Company.
3. Atwater, W. A.: Bulletin 28, United States Department of Agriculture.
4. Eijkman, C.: Arch. f. Hyg., 1906, lviii, 150.
    Arch. path. Anat., 1897, cxlviii, 523.
5. Henriques and Hansen: Zeitschr. für physiol. chem., 1905, xliii, 417.
6. Willcock, E. G., and Hopkins, F. G.: Jour. Physiol., 1906, xxxv, 88.
7. Wisc. Agric. Expt. Sta., Research Bull., No. 17 (1911).
8. McCollum, E. V., and Davis, M.: Jour. Biol. Chem., 1913, xv, 167.
9. Stepp, W.: Biochem. Ztschr., 1909, xxii, 452; Ztschr. f. Biol., 1912, lvii, 135; Ibid, 1912–1913, lix, 366.
10. Hopkins, F. G.: Jour. Physiol., 1912, xliv, 425.
11. Funk, C.: Lancet, London, 1911, ii, 1266.
12. Fraser, H., and Stanton, A. T.: Lancet, London, March 12, 1910, 733; The Etiology of Beri-Beri, Study 12, from the Institute for Medical Research, Federated Malay States, 1911.
13. McCollum and Davis: Jour. Biol. Chem., 1915, xxiii, 247; McCollum, E. V., Simmonds, N., and Pitz, W.: Ibid, 1916, xxv, 105.
14. Funk and Macallum: Jour. Biol. Chem., 1915, xxiii, 419.
15. Henry, W. A.: Wisconsin Agric. Expt. Sta., Annual Report, 1889, 15.

16. Funk, C.: J. State Med., 1912, xx, 341; Biochem. Bull., 1915, iv, 304.
17. McCollum and Davis: Jour. Biol. Chem., 1915, xxiii, 181.
18. McCollum and Davis: Jour. Biol. Chem., 1915, xxiii, 231.
19. McCollum, E. V., and Kennedy, C.: Jour. Biol. Chem., 1916, xxiv, 491.
20. Osborne, T. B., and Mendel, L. B.: Jour. Biol. Chem., 1913, xvi, 431.

CHAPTER II

1. McCollum, Simmonds and Pitz: Jour. Biol. Chem., 1917, xxix, 341.
2. Smith, Theobold: Bureau of Animal Industry, Bacilli in Swine Disease, 1895–1896, 172.
3. Holst, A., and Frölich, T.: Z. Hyg. u. Infektionskrankh, 1913, lxxv, 334.
4. McCollum and Pitz: Jour. Biol. Chem., 1917, xxxi, 229.
5. McCollum and Simmonds: Jour. Biol. Chem., 1917, xxxii, 181.
6. McCollum and Simmonds: Jour. Biol. Chem., 1918, xxxiii, 55.
7. Hart, E. B., McCollum, E. V., Steenbock, H., and Humphery, G. C.: Wisc. Agric. Expt. Sta. Research Bull., 17, 1911.
   Hart and McCollum: Jour. Biol. Chem., 1914, xix, 373.
   McCollum and Davis: Jour. Biol. Chem., 1915, xxi, 615.
   McCollum, Simmonds and Pitz: Ibid, 1916–1917, xxviii, 211.
8. Hart and McCollum: Jour. Biol. Chem., 1914, xix, 373.
   McCollum, Simmonds and Pitz: Ibid, 1916, xxviii, 153.
9. McCollum, E. V., Simmonds, N., and Parsons, H. T.: Unpublished data.
10. McCollum, E. V.: Jour. Am. Med. Assn., 1917, lxviii, 1379.
    Harvey Lecture Series 1916–1917—also—Unpublished data.

11. McCollum, Simmonds and Pitz: Jour. Biol. Chem., 1917, xxix, 521.
12. McCollum, Simmonds and Pitz: Jour. Biol. Chem., 1917, xxx, 13.

Chapter III

1. Slonaker, J. R.: Leland Stanford Junior University, Pub. Univ. Series, 1912.
2. McCollum, Simmonds and Pitz: Jour. Biol. Chem., 1917, xxx, 13.
3. McCollum, Simmonds and Pitz: Am. Jour. Physiol., 1916, xliv, 333.
4. Evvard, J. M.: Proc. Iowa Acad. Sci., 1915, xxii, 375.
5. Loeb, J.: The Dynamics of Living Matter, New York, 1906.
6. Howell, W. H.: Am. Jour. Physiol., 1899, ii, 47; 1902, vi, 181.

Chapter IV

1. McCollum, E. V.: Jour. Biol. Chem., 1914, xix, 323.
2. McCollum and Simmonds: Jour. Biol. Chem., 1917, xxxii, 347.
3. McCollum and Davis: Jour. Biol. Chem., 1915, xx, 415.
4. McCollum, Simmonds and Parsons: Unpublished data.

Chapter V

1. McCollum and Kennedy: Jour. Biol. Chem., 1916, xxiv, 491.
2. Osborne and Mendel: Jour. Biol. Chem., 1913, xvi, 431.
3. McCollum and Simmonds: Jour. Biol. Chem., 1917, xxxii, 347.
4. McCollum, Simmonds and Parsons: Unpublished data.
5. Herdlika, A.: Bulletin 34, Bureau of American Ethnology.

6. Mori, M.: Jahrb. Kinderheilk, 1904, lix, 175.

7. Bloch, C. E.: Ugeskruft für Laeger, 1917, lxxix, 349, cited from Jour. Am. Med. Assn., 1917, lxviii, 1516.

8. Czerny, A. and Keller, A.: Des Kindes, Leipsic, 1906, pt. 2, 67.

9. Little, A. D.: Jour. Am. Med. Assn., 1912, lviii, 2029.

10. Walcott, A. M.: Jour. Am. Med. Assn., 1915, lxv, 2145.

11. Eijkman, C.: Arch. f. Hyg., 1906, lviii, 150.
    Arch. Path. Anat., 1897, cxlviii, 523.

12. Funk, C.: Lancet, London, 1911, ii, 1266.

13. Funk and Macallum: Jour. Biol. Chem., 1915, xxiii, 419.

14. Williams, R. R.: Jour. Biol. Chem., 1916, xxv, 437; 1916, xxvi, 431; 1917, xxix, 495.

15. Jackson, L., and Moore, J. J.: Jour. Infect. Dis., 1916, xix, 478.

16. McCollum and Pitz: Jour. Biol. Chem., 1917, xxxi, 229.

17. Hess, A. F.: Am. Jour. Dis. of Children, 1917, xiv, 337.

18. Goldberger, Joseph: Jour. Am. Med. Assn., 1916, lxvi, 471.

19. Jobling, J. W., and Peterson, W.: Jour. Infect. Dis., 1916, xviii, 501.

20. Thompson-MacFadden Commission, Siler, J. F., Garrison, P. E., and McNeal, W. J.: Archiv. Int. Med. Oct. 1914, p. 453; Journ. Amer. Med. Assn. Sept. 26, 1914, p. 1090.

21. Goldberger, Joseph: Public Health Reports, November 17, 1916, pp. 3159–3173.

22. Goldberger, Joseph: Public Health Reports, Nov. 12, 1915, p. 3.

23. Chittenden, R. H., and Underhill, F. P.: Am. Jour. Physiol., 1917, xliv, 13.

24. McCollum, Simmonds and Parsons: Jour. Biol. Chem., 1918, xxxiii, 411.

25. McCollum and Simmonds: Jour. Biol. Chem., 1917, xxxii, 29.

26. Hess, A. F.: Jour. Am. Med. Assn., 1918, lxx, 900.

CHAPTER VI

1. McCollum and Simmonds: Am. Jour. Phys., 1918, xlvi, 275.
   McCollum, Simmonds and Pitz: Jour. Biol. Chem., 1916, xxvii, 33.
2. Osborne and Mendel: Jour. Biol. Chem., 1915, xx, 379.
3. Andrews, V. L.: Philippine Jour. Science, Series B, 1912, vii, 67.
4. Babcock, S. M.: Twenty-Second Annual Report of Wisconsin Experiment Station, 1905, 129.
5. Eckles, C. H., and Palmer, L. S.: Missouri Agric. Expt. Station Research Bull., 25, 1916.
6. Ducaisne, E.: Gaz. Med., Paris, 1871, 317.

CHAPTER VII

1. Osborne and Mendel: Jour. Biol. Chem., 1915, xx, 381.
2. McCollum and Davis: Jour. Biol. Chem., 1915, xxiii, 247.
3. McCollum, Simmonds and Pitz: Jour. Biol. Chem., 1917, xxix, 521.
4. Sullivan, M. X., and Voegtlin, C.: Jour. Biol. Chem., 1916, xxiv, xvi.
5. Simpson and Edie: 1911–12, Ann. Trop. Med. and Parasit., v, 321.
   Ohler: Jour. Med. Research, 1914, xxxi, 239.
6. Withers and Carruth: Jour. Agric. Research, 1915, v, 261.
   Jour. Biol. Chem., 1917, xxxii, 245.
7. McCollum and Davis: Jour. Biol. Chem., 1915, xxiii, 231.
8. McCollum and Simmonds: 1917, xxxii, 181.

INDEX

Alfalfa flour, 41, 167, 169, 179
Alkaloids, 4
Amino-acids, 5, 74, 75
Appetite, importance of in the selection of food, 64

Barley, 38
Bean, navy, 38, 181
Bean, soy, 38, 175
Beri-beri, 7, 20, 28, 83, 90
Biological method for the analysis of food-stuffs, 20, 21, 56, 113, 161
Butter fat, 16, 89

Carnivora, dietary habits of, 78
Cereal grains, 157, 161
Chittenden and Underhill, studies of pellagra, 107
Corn, 10, 173
Cotton seed flour, 142, 143

Deficiency diseases, 83–87, 91 95, 114
Diet and disease, 6, 7
Diet, essential factors in, 31
Diet of nursing mother in relation to the quality of her milk, 116–129, 185–189
Diet, planning of adequate, 130
Diet, monotonous, 7
Dietary essentials, nomenclature of unidentified, 32

Dietary essentials, chemically unidentified, 23, 34, 47
Dietary habits, 139
Diets from single plant sources, 10
Diets, simplified, 9, 14, 15, 16, 19, 155
Disease and diet, 6, 30, 36, 87, 95, 103, 139
Diseases, deficiency, 83–87, 91, 95, 114

Eggs, 80
Eijkman, 7
Evvard, studies on appetite, 64

Fats, 2, 3, 4
Fats, butter, 16
Fats, egg yolk, 16
Fats, lard, 16
Fats, vegetable, 16
Fat-soluble A, 23, 34, 47, 89, 145, 155
Flax seed, 38
Food analysis, 5
Foods, effect of cooking on, 135–138
Foods, physical properties of, 15
Foods, protective, 82, 141, 147, 149
Foods-stuffs, biological analysis of, 20, 21, 56

197

Food-stuffs, supplementary re-
    lationships among, 61, 71, 81
Fraser and Stanton, 19
Fruits, 7, 142
Funk, 19

Gelatin, 171
Glandular organs, 79
Gliadin, 8
Goldberger, studies of pellagra,
    105–107
Growth, impetus to, 72

Henriques and Hansen, stud-
    ies of simplified diets, 8
Hess, studies of scurvy, 100
Holst, studies of scurvy, 34
Hopkins, studies of simplified
    diets, 18
Hormones, 85

Inorganic salts, importance of,
    4, 22
Iron, 69

Jobling and Peterson, studies
    of pellagra, 105–106

Kafir corn, 38

Leaf, dietary properties of, the,
    41, 44, 53, 77
Leaf and seed mixtures, dietary
    properties of, 61, 167
Lipoids, 3, 17

Meats, 6, 8, 76
Milk, 6, 8, 76
Milk, place of in the diet, 150–
    153

Milk, production, 12
Milk, quality of, as influenced
    by diet, 116–129, 185–189
Millet seed, 38, 175, 177
Muscle tissue, 6, 8, 76
Nomenclature of the chemically
    unidentified dietary essentials,
    84

Osborne and Mendel, 87

Pasteurization of milk, 100–103
Peanut, 142
Peas, 38, 177, 181
Pellagra, 7, 30, 103
Pellagra-producing diets, 108
Polyneuritis, 19, 20, 28
Potato, proteins of, 135, 181
Proteins, 2, 3, 4, 5
Proteins, biological values of,
    5, 24, 74, 75
Proteins, quality not shown by
    chemical analysis, 113

Rat, domestic, 14
Rat, domestic, growth of, 14
Rat, reproduction in, 14
Rice, dietary properties of, 27,
    38, 159, 161
Rickets, 111
Roots, edible, 47
Rye, dietary properties of, 38,
    175

Salts, 4
Scurvy, 7, 30, 34, 36, 37, 95–103
Seed, biological properties of, 53
Seed, and leaf mixtures, dietary
    properties of, 61

Seeds, dietary properties of, 6, 165

Slonaker, studies of vegetarian diet, 57

Smith, Theobald, scurvy in the guinea pig, 34

Sodium, lack of sufficient, in seeds, 23, 49

Starch, 2, 3, 4

Stepp, studies of dietary properties of lipoids, 17

Thompson-McFadden Commission, studies of pellagra, 106

Tubers, dietary properties of, 6, 45

Unidentified factors in the diet, 17, 18

Variety not a safeguard in nutrition, 66

Vegetable oils, 16

Vegetables, 6, 7

Vegetarian diet, 50, 53

Water, 4

Water-soluble B, 29, 34, 47, 155

Wheat and other cereals compared, 139

Wheat, dietary properties of, 10, 20, 21, 38, 157, 159, 171, 175, 179

Wheat flour, bolted, 140

Wheat flour, whole, 140

Xerophthalmia of dietary origin, 87, 139

Printed in the United States of America

THE following pages contain advertisements of
books by the same author or on kindred subjects

Organic Chemistry for Medical Students

By ELMER V. McCOLLUM, Ph.D.
Professor of Bio-Chemistry, Johns Hopkins Medical School

Illustrated. Cloth, 12mo. $2.25

The author has based this work on the new biological methods of teaching chemistry to medical students. The work is developed from Dr. McCollum's unusual researches and experiments and the subject matter is presented with great clearness and attention to teaching principles. It is unique in scope and methods and is designed for the use of both medical and pre-medical students.

———

THE MACMILLAN COMPANY
Publishers   64-66 Fifth Avenue   New York

Chemistry of Food and Nutrition

New and Revised Edition

By HENRY C. SHERMAN

Professor of Food Chemistry in Columbia
University

$2.00

This new edition, entirely rewritten and enlarged to nearly twice the original size, incorporates the recent advances in all of the topics considered in the previous edition as well as some new topics which have lately become important to the student of food and nutrition.

The review of the chemistry of the organic foodstuffs considered in the first edition in one chapter is now treated in three chapters and contains considerable matter of distinctly nutritional import. The chapters on digestion, metabolism, food requirements, dietary standards and economic use of food have all been rewritten and expanded to embrace recent advances. New chapters on the specific relations of food to growth and on the so-called deficiency diseases and vitamine theories have been added.

THE MACMILLAN COMPANY

Publishers   64–66 Fifth Avenue   New York

Some Aspects of Food Economy

By MARY S. ROSE

Everyday Foods in War Time $.80

This little book was written in response to a request for "a war message about food." It gives a simple explanation of the part which some of our common foods play in our diet, and points out how the necessary saving of fat, fuel, sugar, and meat can be made without a loss of health or strength.

There are chapters on the Milk Pitcher in the Home; Cereals We Ought to Eat; Meats We Ought to Save; The Potato and Its Substitutes; Are Fruits and Vegetables Luxuries? Sugar and Spice and Everything Nice; On Being Economical and Patriotic at the Same Time.

Feeding the Family $2.10

This is a clear concise account in simple everyday terms of the ways in which modern knowledge of the science of nutrition may be applied in ordinary life. The food needs of the members of the typical family group—men, women, infants, children of various ages—are discussed in separate chapters, and many illustrations in the form of food plans and dietaries are included. The problems of the housewife in trying to reconcile the needs of different ages and tastes at the same table are also taken up, as are the cost of food and the construction of menus. A final chapter deals with feeding the sick.

THE MACMILLAN COMPANY

Publishers   64–66 Fifth Avenue   New York

War Bread

By ALONZO E. TAYLOR

Professor of Physiological Chemistry, University of Pennsylvania; member of the United States Food Administration

$.60

Dr. Taylor states that it is his purpose to make clear just what must be accomplished in order that we may give to every member of the allied people his full share in our pooled food stuff at the lowest comparable cost and with the least labor. With this in view, he takes up the following topics:

What the Allies Need; What We Possess; Why We are Limited in Wheat; Food Value of the Different Grains; Ways of Stretching Wheat; and Waste of Wheat.

The Food Problem

By VERNON KELLOGG and ALONZO E. TAYLOR

With an Introduction by Herbert Hoover

$1.25

"Food," says Mr. Hoover in his introduction, "is always a problem in every phase of its production, handling, and consumption. It is a problem with every farmer, every transporter and seller, every state and nation. And now very conspicuously it is a problem with three great groups; namely, the Allies, the Central Empires, and the Neutrals; in a word, it is a great international problem."

Some of the questions which the book considers in detail are: What is the problem in detail? What are the general conditions of its solution? What are the immediate problems and particulars which concern us? and finally, What are we actually doing to meet the problem?

THE MACMILLAN COMPANY

Publishers   64–66 Fifth Avenue   New York

WS - #0040 - 130121 - C0 - 229/152/13 - PB - 9781330356593 - Gloss Lamination